Defeat BLOOD PRESSURE with Alternative Therapies

Includes

- Homeopathy • Herbal Remedies • Ayurveda
- Chinese Herbs • Acupuncture • Acupressure
- Yoga • Exercises • Juice Therapy • Diet & Nutrition • Home Remedies • Biofeedback
- Aromatherapy • Massage

Blood Pressure and Its

- Causes • Signs & Symptoms • Lab Investigations
- Complications of Blood Pressure
- Management of Special Cases • Prevention

Dr. Ritu Jain
BHMS

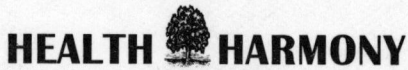

HEALTH HARMONY
An imprint of
B. Jain Publishers (P) Ltd.
An ISO 9001 : 2000 Certified Company
USA — EUROPE — INDIA

DEFEAT BLOOD PRESSURE WITH ALTERNATIVE THERAPIES

First Edition: 2008

All rights reserved. No part of this book may be reproduced, stored in a retrieval system or transmitted, in any form or by any means, mechanical, photocopying, recording or otherwise, without any prior written permission of the publisher.

© with the publishers

Published by Kuldeep Jain for
HEALTH HARMONY
An imprint of
B. Jain Publishers (P) Ltd.
An ISO 9001 : 2000 certified Company
1921/10, Chuna Mandi, Paharganj, New Delhi 110 055 (INDIA)
Tel.: 91-11-2358 0800, 2358 1100, 2358 1300, 2358 3100
Fax: 91-11-2358 0471 *Email:* info@bjain.com
Website: www.bjainbooks.com

Printed in India by
J.J. Offset Printers
522, FIE, Patpar Ganj, Delhi - 110 092
Tel.: 91-11-2216 9633, 2215 6128

ISBN: 978-81-319-0336-0

*This Book is Dedicated
to
My Caring Husband
Rohit Jain*

Publisher's Note

In today's time, lifestyle disorders have become a part of our lives. But this scenario needs to be changed and we need to put a check before it's too late. One of the ways is to increase awareness about the prevention of lifestyle disorders, their causes and the treatment options available.

To tackle this epidemic of lifestyle disorders we as a publisher are always trying to publish books which can help in dissemination of knowledge about lifestyle disorders. We are proud to come out with this third book of **'Defeat Series'** in which we are covering various diseases and their management.

Defeat Blood Pressure with Alternative Therapies deals with all the aspects of blood pressure from its causes, symptomatology, investigations required, and above all a detailed information on its management. All treatment options available, from the conventional medicine to different alternative therapies, have been included.

We hope that all our readers would find this book beneficial for themselves as well as their families.

Kuldeep Jain
CEO, B. Jain Publishers

Preface

My purpose of writing this series is to provide information on homeopathy as well as some other alternative therapies to general public and their uses in particular health disorders like joint pains, diabetes, high blood pressure, back pain, constipation, headaches and migraine and so on.

People now wish to take more responsibility for their own health. An increasing number of people want to understand how to prevent illness and, if they do become ill, then to understand the causes and determine how they can help themselves recover. Homeopathy offers a simple, effective, extremely safe, and relatively inexpensive way of accomplishing this – provided it is practiced with common sense.

By understanding basics of homeopathy one will be able to take better care of his physical, mental and emotional well-being. This book aims to clear mysteries surrounding homeopathy and would help in making an informed choice about homeopathic self-treatment.

However, it is my kind request that under no circumstances, patients suffering from serious ailments (or those uncertain of their ailment) should consider self-treatment. They should always consult a well-qualified experienced homeopathic physician.

Highlights of the book are as follows:

- Information on homeopathy – All the questions have been answered that you always wanted to ask. This would help you understand the basics of homeopathy and integrate it into your healthcare.

- Many figures, diagrams and illustrations have been included to make the topic interesting and easy to understand
- Every aspect of blood pressure has been explained in easy-to-understand language – structure and functioning of heart, causes, signs and symptoms, when to consult your doctor, lab investigations, treatments, complications and prevention.
- Complication of blood pressure have been explained with their causes, signs and symptoms, lab investigations, treatment, management and prevention.
- Allopathic treatment has been dealt comprehensively in a separate chapter.
- Under homeopathic treatment, only those remedies which have been found very effective in a particular disorder have been listed with their indicated symptoms and dosages. This makes the choice of remedy very effortless.
- In addition to homeopathic treatment the following complementary therapies have been included:
  - Yoga
  - Exercise
  - Herbal remedies
  - Home remedies
  - Chinese medicine
  - Ayurveda
  - Acupuncture
  - Acupressure
  - Juice therapy
  - Diet & nutrition
  - Biofeedback

- Aromatherapy
- Massage

- With the help of the above-mentioned additional information, the patient can complement the homeopathic treatment with other suitable therapies to get maximum benefit in shortest time.
- Management of following special cases have been dealt in a separate chapter.
  - Pregnancy and high blood pressure
  - Oral contraceptive and high blood pressure
  - Elderly people and high blood pressure
  - Children and high blood pressure

Above all, as one works his way through this book, he gets a message and a ray of hope. Whether the disorder is recent or lifelong, this book presents with treatments that are based on research, evidence and experience. They work and they will work for you. All the best with your journey. Now it's the time to begin...

Dr. Ritu Jain

Acknowledgments

I would never have started writing these books if Dr. Rohit Jain, my husband, would not have encouraged me to do so and then encouraged and supported me along the way – thanks Rohit! Also how could I forget my lovely daughter, Adya who kept me refreshed with her innocent activities.

My indebtness to my parents Shri P.K. Shrivastava and Smt. Malti Shrivastava for their constant help and motivation.

I am also thankful to Dr. Vimal K. Bhardwaj for beautifully drawing the diagrams of the book.

My thanks also to my publisher, Mr. Kuldeep Jain, who approached me to put my knowledge together in form of a book.

I'm sincerely grateful to my patients who have enriched my experience and confidence over the years. And to my brother, sisters, their families, and my friends for their inspiration and support.

References

While no reference has been made to authors through the work owing to the writer's desire to economize space, yet she desires to express her indebtness to the numerous writers upon these subjects as they have each been freely consulted in the preparation of this work.

About the Author

Dr. Ritu Jain is a BHMS (Bachelor of Homeopathic Medicine and Surgery) with honors. She also has a BSc (Gold Medalist) in Life Sciences. As a student, she was among the top few in both academic accomplishments as well as extra curricular activities. For the last 11 years she is healing people along with her husband Dr. Rohit Jain, at Vital Force Homeopathic Clinic. She is also a Member of VHAD (Voluntary Health Association of Delhi) which keeps her busy providing health services to the underprivileged. Her patients recognize her as a tolerant listener and compassionate physician. She uses multi-disciplinary approach of complementary therapies to treat the "whole" person. She has written 2 other books on homeopathy and alternative therapies, namely, **Defeat Joint Pains with Alternative Therapies** and **Defeat Diabetes with Alternative Therapies**. At present she is working on her next book.

Recognized as an expert in solving complex cases of skin, infertility and female gynecological ailments, Dr. Ritu's line of treatment includes her own special homeopathic preparations. Elaborating on her practice Dr. Ritu says, "Homeopathy emphasizes on using a revolutionary and holistic approach to eliminate the root cause of the disease. It is not only safe, but also effective. It adopts a highly sophisticated and scientific approach to health, disease and treatment." Dr. Ritu says that homeopathy offers the most safe and natural solution to chronic diseases such as respiratory problems, abdominal, skin and psychiatric disorders.

CONTENTS

Publisher's Note v
Preface vi
Acknowledgements xi
References xii
About the Author xi

CHAPTERS

1. **Information on Homeopathy** 1
   - Questions you always wanted to ask... 1
2. **Introduction to Blood Pressure** 11
3. **Structure and Function of Heart** 13
   - Blood Circulation 13
   - Heart and its Chambers 14
   - Heart Valves and Circulation of Blood 15
   - Blood Circulation (Pulmonary and
     Systemic Circulation) 17
   - Heart Sounds 20
4. **Blood Pressure** 23
   - Normal Values of Blood Pressure 24
   - Control of Blood Pressure 25
   - Conditions Affecting Blood Pressure 29
5. **High Blood Pressure** 33
   - Affects of High Blood Pressure 34
   - Types of High Blood Pressure 36
   - Low Blood Pressure 39
6. **Causes** 41
7. **Symptoms** 51
8. **Diagnosis and Investigations** 55

- Sphygmomanometer 55
- Measuring Blood Pressure 58
- Investigations 66
- Interview (Sample) 68
- Physical Examination 70

9. **Management of High Blood Pressure** **77**
   - Aims of Treatment 77
10. **Treatment without Drugs** **79**
    - Diet (or Healthy Eating) 80
    - Weight Control 96
    - Exercise 103
    - Smoking 106
11. **Treatment with Drugs** **109**
    - Treatment with Allopathy Drugs 110
    - Goal of Treatment 110
    - Controlling Blood Pressure by Drugs 111
12. **Homeopathic Treatment** **135**
13. **Other Alternative Therapies** **159**
    - Acupressure 160
    - Chinese Herbalism 161
    - Juice Therapy 163
    - Herbal Therapy 165
    - Body Massage 168
    - Yoga 169
    - Aromatherapy 171
    - Breathing and Relaxation 176
    - Mind and Spirit Therapies 179
    - Meditation 180
    - Hypnosis 184
    - Home Remedies 185
14. **Special Considerations** **189**
    - Pregnancy 189
    - Oral Contraceptive 196

- Elderly People 198
- Children 200
- Diabetes 201
- Asthma and other Chest Disease 205
- High Blood Cholesterol Level 207

15. Long-term Complications 209
- Heart and Aorta 209
- Brain 210
- Legs and Feet 211
- Eyes 211
- Kidneys 211
- Other Parts of the Body 211
- Angina 211
- Heart Attack 213
- Stroke 215

Chapter 1

Information on Homeopathy

QUESTIONS YOU ALWAYS WANTED TO ASK...

By understanding the basics, one would be able to take more responsibility for his own health.

What is homeopathy?

Homeopathy, a therapeutic system used for over 250 years, works on the principle of "like cures like"—an illness is treated with a substance which could produce similar symptoms in a healthy person. However, homeopathic medicines are given in highly diluted forms and are therefore extremely safe and have no side-effects.

Homeopathy is a holistic system of treatment. It aims to treat the whole person, rather than just the physical symptoms.

What is a homeopathic consultation like?

The homeopath will ask not only about ones illness but also about the way he is affected by environmental factors such as temperature and the weather, what kinds of food he eats or avoids, his moods and feelings as well as his medical history in order to establish a complete picture. This is then related to the description of your current symptoms in order to prescribe the correct remedy at the right strength. Whereas in allopathic medical practice, people diagnosed with the same condition will generally be given the same medicine.

Every individual reacts and adapts in a different way to their surroundings and this is accepted and respected in homeopathy for remedy selection. The way people adapt to new home, family, or work environment; their reaction to external circumstances; their past and present experiences; and their general state of mind are all key attributes of patient's assessment and treatment.

What happens in subsequent consultations?

The subsequent consultations entail discussions about what has happened to the particular symptom(s) - are there changes in intensity or frequency, has the patient noticed any changes in his/her general health (appetite, sleep, bowel habit, etc.). To a homeopath, this most recent picture is again a new symptom totality that needs to be assessed; the medicines are again prescribed taking this changing totality into consideration.

The second prescription is therefore based on the new symptom totality - which may also change from patient to patient, even in cases where the diagnosis of the disorder might be similar. In homeopathy there are no fixed rules for describing a particular 'plan of treatment' for a particular disorder - the doctor would prescribes on the basis of totality of the symptoms, the changes and adjustments are made according to changes reported by the patient.

What is constitutional treatment in homeopathy?

According to homeopathy, mind and body are very much linked and physical problems cannot be effectively cured without understanding and putting right the person's constitution and character. Constitution in homeopathy means a person's state of health, including their temperament and any inherited and acquired characteristics. As loads of aspects of human being contribute to constitution therefore a homeopath usually asks many questions before he could from the constitution of a person.

Homeopathy believes that if the constitution of a person is healthy, he will not succumb to any infection, i.e. bacteriae and viruses will not affect him as his susceptibility is low. This is the basic difference between allopathy and homeopathy. Allopaths believe that one becomes sick due to infection, i.e. bacteriae and viruses; hence their treatment is aimed at killing the infection using strong drugs. This however, further reduces the immunity of the person, making it weaker and the person becomes more susceptible and falls sick again and again. Homeopaths, however, believe that first the constitution becomes weak and then the individual becomes susceptible to infection. The bacteriae and viruses are the end products of disease process and not the cause of disease. The bacteriae and viruses are everywhere; they will not affect you till your immunity is strong. In homeopathy, treatment is aimed at raising the vitality, i.e. immunity of the person so that he can fight with the diseases himself. This is why homeopathy is able to cure permanently while in allopathy there are frequent remissions.

Individualistic nature of homeopathic prescription

Unlike allopathy, homeopathy serves to individual's needs. Therefore, in homeopathy two people are unlikely to be prescribed the same remedy. One remedy may be prescribed constitutionally for general bodily imbalances and another remedy may be prescribed simultaneously for specific, acute symptoms. On the subsequent visit the remedies may be changed depending upon the progress of the patient.

How does a homeopath chooses the potency, i.e. strength of the remedy?

Several factors are considered while deciding the potency of the remedy prescribed like, condition to be treated, the strength of the patient, the age of the patient, and the circumstances. Not only must the remedy given be suitable, but the potency chosen must also be appropriate to the individual patient.

What reactions should one expect after taking a homeopathic remedy?

Usually after taking a well-indicated homeopathic medicine, the person feels better in all aspects – physical, mental and emotional. Occasionally after taking a homeopathic medicine the existing symptoms may worsen slightly. This effect will be brief and is a good sign that the body's natural healing energies have started to counteract the illness. After this, the symptoms will subside and health will be regained. If symptoms do not go away, consult the homeopath.

Taking homeopathic remedies . . .

- Avoid eating for half-an-hour before or after taking the medicine. This is because homeopathic medicines get absorbed from the inner linings of the mouth. Substances usually leave a coating in the oral cavity and also an odor. This may hinder the absorption of the medicine. However water can be taken.

- It is also advisable to completely avoid strong substances like coffee and mint while taking homeopathic remedies because these may antidote the remedy prescribed

- Touching medicines may inactivate them, therefore, avoid touching homeopathic remedies. It is best to tip 4 pills into the lid of the container and then tip the medicine into your mouth. If the pills are touched or dropped, they should not be returned to the container. Otherwise the remedy may lose its power.

- Remedies should be stored away from strong light, strong temperature variations and strong smells

Can homeopathic medicines be taken along with allopathic medicines?

Homeopathic medicines can be safely taken along with other

allopathic medicines of blood pressure and diabetes medicines. Allopathic medicines are not stopped immediately and your homeopath will reduce the other drugs if health begins to improve under the influence of the homeopathic remedies.

Origin of homeopathy and its present status

The founder of homeopathy, Dr. Samuel Christian Hahnemann, MD, was a German allopathic doctor of his time. He was disatisfied with his profession and left his career in allopathic medicine to research alternative treatments. He began treating patients with a principle of "like cures like". He called his new system "homeopathy", from the Greek word: *homeo* meaning "similar" and *pathos* meaning "suffering."

Government of India through Central Council of Homeopathy controls and reviews education, research and practice of homeopathy in India. In India most of the government run clinics and hospitals have a homeopathic unit.

Homeopathy in India is a full-fledged Bachelor's degree course spanning 5½ years of training with one year internship and a postgraduate MD course. There are around 147 homeopathic medical colleges all over India which offer undergraduate medical education; many of these are government run while others are run by private educational societies. Out of these 23 offer postgraduate education. Minimum qualification for admission into these colleges is high school with Biology, Physics and Chemistry as majors. The students also have to undergo an entrance exam for admission into the undergraduate homeopathy degree course. The above process ensures that only the talented students become future homeopaths.

There is no difference between the homeopathic medical curricula and that of MBBS. In 4½ years the students learn Anatomy, Physiology, Biochemistry, Microbiology, Pathology, Parasitology, Forensic Medicine, Gynecology, Obstetrics, Ophthalmology, ENT, Surgery, Community Medicine, Practice of Medicine along with Homeopathic Pharmacy, Repertory, Materia Medica and

Homeopathic Philosophy. From the second year on, they learn bedside medicine and attend clinical classes. Exams are conducted at the end the academic year. At the end of 4½ years, after passing their final exams, they are awarded the BHMS degree (Bachelor of Homeopathic Medicine and Surgery).

There is a 1 year internship after that where the prospective homeopaths are posted in the hospital and other clinics which are operated by government. At the end of the internship, the homeopaths register themselves with the State Homeopathy Board which in effect is a license to practise.

There are postgraduate courses also. Admission to these is through an entrance exam.

Why homeopathic medicines are slow acting?

Homeopathy is NOT slow acting. This myth is popular, because most of the people approaching homeopathy have a long history of chronic ailments, and hence the treatment takes time. Since homeopathy offers a much better alternative than allopathy in such ailments, it is believed that homeopathy is slow acting. Homeopathy is, in fact, FAST and RAPID in its action in acute conditions.

How effective are homeopathic medicines?

The efficacy and effectiveness of homeopathic medicines has been demonstrated by more than 250 years of successful use by physicians all over the globe. It is the better and sometimes the only alternative in many ailments. Homeopathy cures curable conditions and palliates incurable conditions.

How can small white pills be effective?

Most of the medicines are prepared in an alcohol base. The white sugar globules or pills are only a medium or vehicle for the transport of the medicine into the body. These doubts arise in people who use homeopathic medicines for the first time. It is the medicine (in liquid form) that acts on the patient.

Homeopathy is nothing, but faith healing?

NO, scientific and random double-blind controlled studies have repeatedly indicated that homeopathy is not placebo effect. The effects of homeopathic medicines have been observed repeatedly on neonates, infants, unconscious patients, animals where faith healing is not possible. Hence, the misbelieve that homeopathy is placebo is nothing but prejudice.

Do homeopathic medicines have any side effects?

No, homeopathic medicines do not have any side effects, as they are administered in minute doses and do not have a chemical or mechanical effect on the body.

How are homeopathic medicines made?

Homeopathic medicines are derived from a variety of natural materials and are prepared in licensed laboratories under strict quality control. They are given in tablet, globules, pills, liquid or powder form and are available in different, but extremely dilute strengths known as potencies.

What is the shelf life of homeopathic medicines?

If properly stored, homeopathic medicines can be used for years without any deterioration of quality.

Storage Guidelines

Medicines are to be kept tightly capped at room temperature in a cool, dry, dust free environment and away from direct sunlight. They should not be exposed to strong odors. Don't store your remedies in your medicine chest if you also keep things like *balm*, or cough drops that contain menthol.

Is homeopathy safe for children and pregnant females?

Yes, homeopathy is totally safe for children. It can also be safely administered to pregnant females.

Can diabetic patients take the sweet sugar pill?

Yes, diabetics can take pills because the amount of sugar present is very minute. Also, medicines can be administered in distilled water, thereby avoiding pills.

Can homeopathy be used in emergencies and is it 'fast acting'?

Yes, homeopathy is effective and efficient in acute conditions and in emergencies. The right remedy in the right potency and the right dose can have amazing action in acute diseases.

What other things promote recovery along with homeopathy?

All homeopathic remedies work best when combined with balanced diet, yoga, a low-stress environment, and emotional and intellectual states that promote a balanced body system.

What are the types of disorders in which homeopathy would benefit?

Usually people are under the impression that homeopathy can treat only chronic diseases like arthritis, skin conditions, migraine, menstrual irregularities, hemorrhoids, digestive conditions, allergies, cancer, liver, kidney, heart and lung disorders. But many people do not know that it is very effective and prompt in acute conditions like tonsillitis, pharyngitis, viral fevers, vomiting, diarrhea, dysentery, asthma, bronchitis, constipation, injury, childhood disorders etc. Sometimes it may cut short the attack of the disease all together and in most cases, gives relief faster than conventional treatment without any side effects.

While on homeopathic treatment if some acute trouble arises; in that case can allopathic treatment be taken along with constitutional homeopathic treatment?

This would depend on the problem you have and your

homeopathic treatment. This issue is best decided by the consulting homeopath.

Is it true that homeopathic medicines are tested on healthy human beings?

Yes, it is a fact that homeopathic medicines are first tested or proved on healthy human beings of both the sexes. The effects are recorded and a compendium of the symptoms/signs is prepared.

Using these compendium as references, a homeopathic physician selects a remedy to be given to a patient.

How far are laboratory investigations useful to a homeopathic physician?

They are useful only to understand whether the case can respond to homeopathy or not, and to decide the prognosis which can only be decided after an exhaustive case taking. These are also necessary to assess the progress of the case.

Can pet animals be treated by homeopathic medicines?

One of the wonderful advantages of using homeopathic medicines is that it is very easy to give them to animals. There's no need to force pills down their throats or squirt nasty-tasting liquids in their mouths. In fact, giving an animal his remedy can be part of a quiet, relaxing healing time for both: master and pet. Just follow these simple steps:

- Before you begin, remember to rinse your hands well to remove any residual odors that might de-potentize your remedies
- If you can handle pet animal comfortably make him relax and spend a few moments stroking and talking to him softly until he relaxes. If possible, make him lie on his side. Make a point of gently touching him around his mouth so that he associates this contact with your loving attention.
- To avoid touching the remedies open he bottle and gently tap

the required globules - usually four - into the cap, returning any extras from the cap back into the vial. If you touch a globule or it falls on the floor, throw it away; returning it to the vial might de-potentize the remaining globules.

- If the patient is a dog, cat, or other small mammal, stroke the side of his face, then gently lift the side of his lip and drop the globules directly from the cap onto his gums. Allow his lip to fall back against the gums and continue to gently stroke his face and body. It is possible that he continues to lie quietly, enjoying the attention and barely noticing the sweet-tasting pills dissolving in his mouth.

- If it's not practical to have the animal lie on his side (as with a horse or other large animal, or one who is a little tense), it's okay to use fingers to place the pills in his mouth. As long as there are no strong smelling substances in the hands, touching the remedy briefly will not de-potentize it. Simply pour the correct number of pills from the vial cap into the palm of one hand, then pick those up with the thumb and forefinger of other hand and place them on the animal's gums, slide them between his lips.

    Ideally, the pellets will dissolve in membranes as they release their healing energy into his system. However, if he chews and swallows the pellets, don't worry. They will still do their job. Even if they remain on his gums for few moments before he spits them out, there's an excellent chance his system will receive the benefit of the healing energy.

- If the animal is unwilling, crush the pellets and dissolve them in a small amount of water and administer it with an eye dropper or offer it for drinking. It's fine if he doesn't gulp all of it up right away. The amount of medicine he received in one dose is unimportant and remaining solution can be disposed off.

■

Chapter 2
Introduction to Blood Pressure

Blood pressure is a major problem in today's high-stress world. It is a silent disease that degrades health and is precursor to serious cardiovascular diseases. High blood pressure is caused by clogging of arteries with fatty deposits, calcium/fiber deficiencies, poor sugar metabolism, obesity and lack of exercise.

Nutritional prevention measures and natural therapies have proved to reduce mortality better than many aggressive medical intervention techniques and advanced drugs. The good news is that diet is also the single most influential factor for preventing these problems. If one changes his lifestyle he can improve his future far more than a lifetime of dependence on drugs.

It may be due to intensive struggle for existence associated with ambition, artificial method of living, continual anxiety, irregular hours, adulterated and unwholesome food, want of faith in religion and many things in particular to modern life undoubtedly play important role in its causation.

The book discusses the key treatment modalities for all types of pressure and offers, diet, allopathy, homeopathy, herbal and unconventional medicine including yoga, pranayam, juice therapy, massage, aromatherapy, meditation, hypnosis and the time tested home remedies. Infact it teaches the method to control blood pressure and live a long and healthy life without any hassles by educating the reader.

In preparing the work, the assistance has been derived from standard works, current literature, private and clinical practice. This book is prepared keeping in view the interests of physician as well as public. Read it carefully then act, do consult a physician as self medication is not advised or encouraged.

Chapter 3
Structure and Function of Heart

Blood pressure is the pressure by which the blood is circulated in blood vessels. The heart is a muscular pump that provides the pressure to move the blood along. Blood vessels have elastic walls and provide some resistance to the flow.

BLOOD CIRCULATION

The function of the blood is to transport material around the body, mainly to take nutrients and oxygen to body cells to keep them alive and well, and to remove their waste products such as carbon dioxide. Blood picks up oxygen in the lungs from the air. This oxygenated blood enters the heart, and is then pumped out to all parts of the body through *arteries* (larger blood vessels). Larger blood vessels branch into smaller and smaller one and then to microscopic *arterioles* which eventually form tiny blood vessels known as *capillaries*. This network allows blood to reach every cell of the body and provide oxygen, which is used by cells. The deoxygenated blood returns to the heart from cells through the blood vessels known as *veins*. This deoxygenated blood is pumped back to the lungs to pick up more oxygen.

HEART AND ITS CHAMBERS

The heart has four chambers. The two superior chambers are the *atria*, and the two inferior chambers are the *ventricle*.

Right Atrium

The right atrium receives blood from three veins: *the superior vena cava, inferior vena cava* and *coronary sinus*. Blood passes from the right atrium into the right ventricle through a valve called the tricuspid valve. It is known as tricuspid because it consists of three leaflets or cusps.

Left Atrium

The left atrium forms most of the base of the heart. It receives blood from the lungs through four *pulmonary veins*. Between the right atrium and left atrium is a thin partition called the *interatrial septum*. Blood passes from the left atrium into the left ventricle through the bicuspid (*mitral*) valve. It is known as bicuspid because it consists of two cusps.

Right Ventricle

The right ventricle is separated from the left ventricle by a partition called the *interventricular septum*. Blood passes from the right ventricle through the *pulmonary valve* into a large artery called the *pulmonary trunk*, which divides into right and left *pulmonary arteries*.

Left Ventricle

Blood passes from the left ventricle through the *aortic valve* into the largest artery of the body, the *aorta*. Some of the blood in

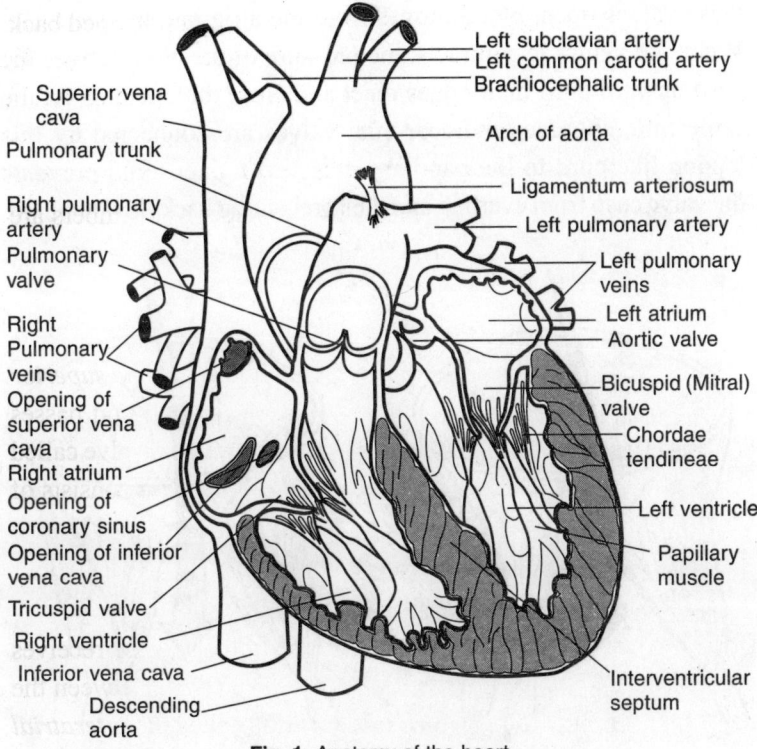

Fig. 1: Anatomy of the heart

the aorta flow into the *coronary arteries*, which carry blood to the heart wall. Branches of the aorta carry blood throughout the body.

HEART VALVES AND CIRCULATION OF BLOOD

Each of the four valves helps to ensure the one way flow of blood. The valves open to let blood flow through and then close to prevent the backflow of blood. Valves open and close in response to pressure changes as the heart contracts and relaxes. As each chamber of the heart contracts, it pushes a volume of blood into a ventricle or out of the heart into an artery.

The tricuspid and bicuspid valves located between an atrium and a ventricle, are termed *atrioventricular* (AV) *valves*. When these valves open, blood moves from the atria into the ventricle. When the ventricle contracts, the pressure of the blood drives the cusp upward until their edges meet and close the opening. At the same time chordae tendineae (the valves are connected by this tendon like cord to the papillary muscles) tightens and prevents the valve cusp from everting and thus preventing back flow of blood.

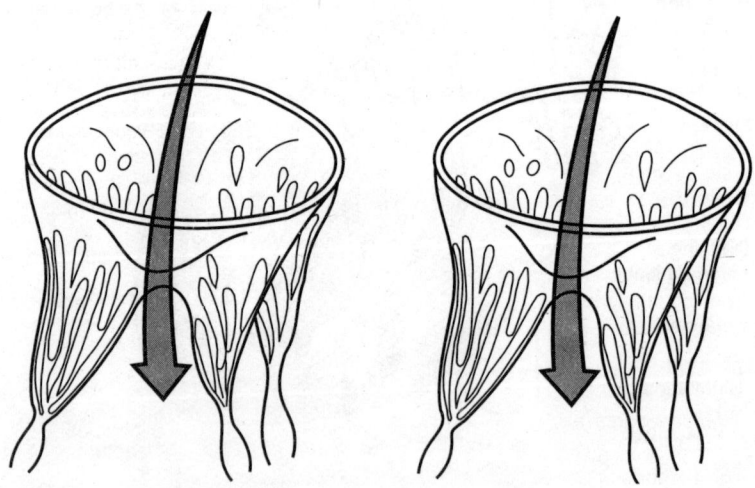

Fig. 2: Heart valves and circulation of blood

The aortic and pulmonary valves are known as the *semilunar* (SL) *valves* because they are made up of three moon-shaped cusps. The SL valves allow ejection of blood from the heart into arteries but prevent backflow of blood into the ventricles. The SL valves open when pressure in the ventricles exceeds the pressure in the arteries, permitting ejection of blood from the ventricles into the pulmonary trunk and aorta. As the ventricles relax, blood starts to flow back towards the heart. As the back flowing blood fills the cusps, the SL valves close.

Valves do not guard the entrance of the vena cava into the atriums.

BLOOD CIRCULATION (PULMONARY AND SYSTEMIC CIRCULATION)

Circulatory system consists of two circular systems, the circulation through lungs, called the *pulmonary circulation* and circulation through the rest of the body called the *systemic circulation*.

Blood flows through these two systems by two pumps, the right and left side of heart. Although these right and left pumps beat together, the blood in each side is entirely separate and to some extend function independently. The left side of heart is bigger, more muscular and carries a much heavier work-load than the right because pushing blood through lungs is much easier than pushing it through every part of body.

The heart pumps blood into two closed circuits. The two circuits are arranged in series – the output of one becomes the input of the other. The left side of the heart is the pump for the entire body (systemic circulation), it receives bright red, oxygen-rich blood from the lungs. The left ventricle pumps blood into the aorta. From

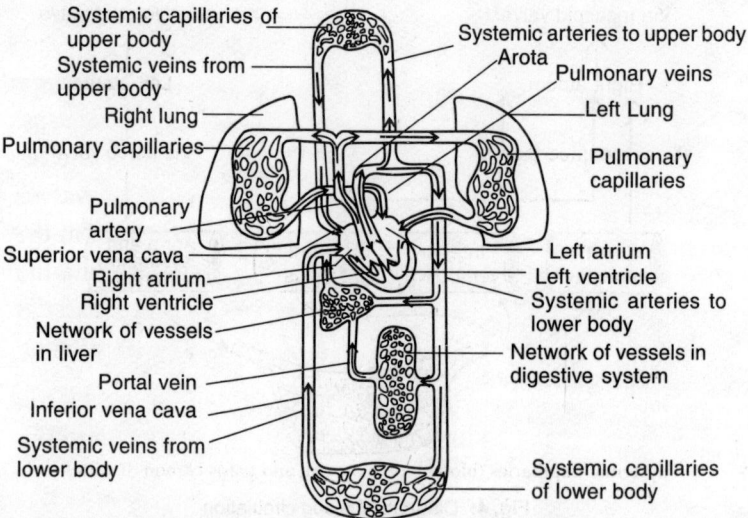

Fig. 3: Diagram showing the circulation of blood

the aorta, the blood flows into smaller systemic arteries that carries blood to all the organs of the body except for air sac (alveoli) of the lungs. In every part of the body arteries finally lead into systemic capillaries where exchange of nutrients and gases occurs. Blood unloads oxygen and picks up carbon dioxide (CO_2). Blood flows

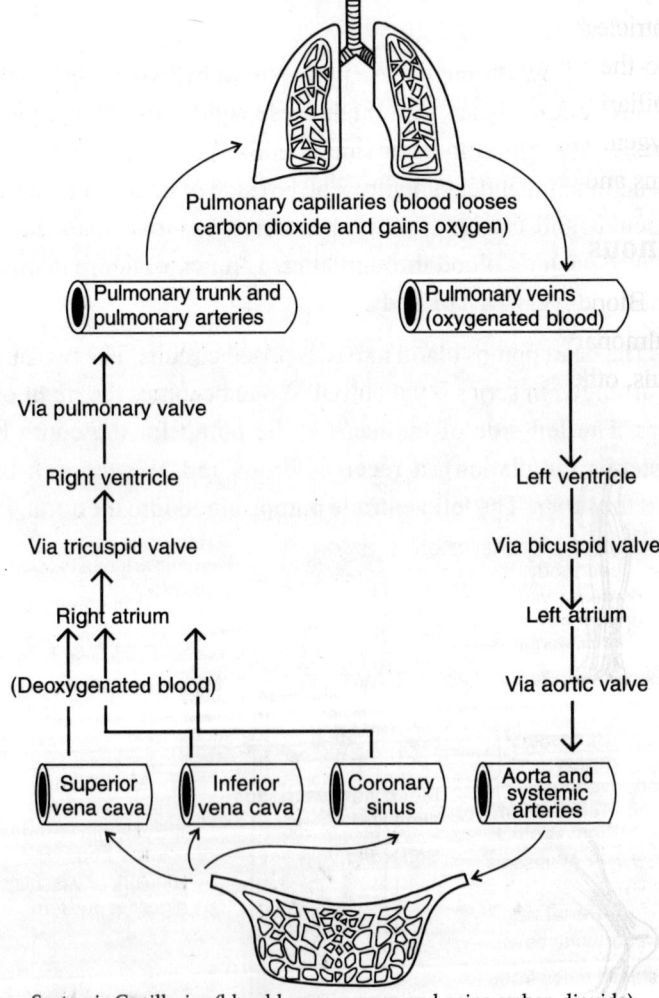

Systemic Capillaries (blood looses oxygen and gains carbon dioxide)

Fig. 4: Diagram of blood circulation

through capillaries and then enters systemic venules. Venules carry deoxygenated blood away from tissues to systemic veins and then back to the right atrium of the heart.

The right side of the heart receives all the dark deoxygenated blood from the systemic circulation. Right side of heart is the pump for pulmonary circulation. Blood flows from right atrium to right ventricle and is then pumped into the pulmonary trunk, which carries it to the right and left lung through pulmonary arteries. In lung capillaries blood unloads CO_2 (which is exhaled), and picks up oxygen. The freshly oxygenated blood then flows into pulmonary veins and returns to the left atrium of the heart.

Venous Return

Blood is under pressure at all points through out both systems (pulmonary and systemic circulation), in arteries, capillaries and veins, otherwise it would not circulate. Pressure in capillaries has

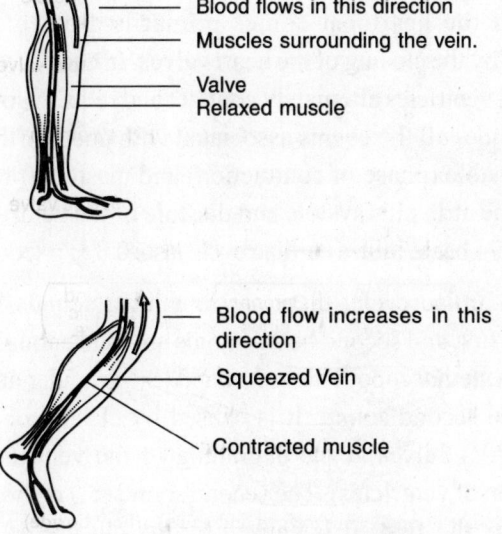

Fig. 5: The muscular pump

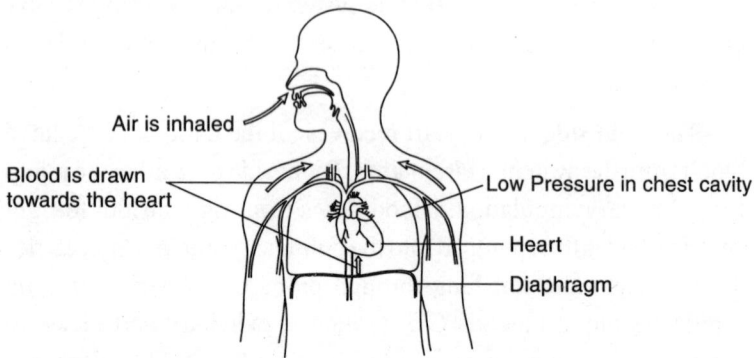

Fig. 6: Inhalation acting as a respiratory pump

to be kept constant, so that the conditions for the transfer of gas and nutrients in body cells and tissues remain unchanged, despite huge differences in what the rest of body may be doing. This is the main reason for the variability of arterial blood pressure.

HEART SOUNDS

The sound of the heartbeat comes primarily from blood turbulence caused by the closing of the heart valves. In each cardiac cycle, the atria and ventricles alternately contract and relax. A single cardiac cycle includes all the events associated with one heartbeat which includes systole (phase of contraction) and diastole (phase of relaxation) of the atria plus systole and diastole of the ventricle. When heart rate is 75 beats/min. a cardiac cycle lasts 0.8 of a second.

During each cardiac cycle, there are four heart sounds, but normally only the first and second heart sounds are loud enough to be heard through a stethoscope. The first sound (S_1) is louder and a bit longer than the second sound. It is caused by closure of the atrioventricular (AV) valves at the beginning of the ventricular systole (contraction of ventricles). The second sound (S_2) is shorter and not as loud as the first. It is caused by the closure of the semilunar (SL) valves at the beginning of the ventricular diastole (relaxation of ventricle). Normally third (S_3) and fourth (S_4) sounds are not loud enough to be heard. S_3 is due to blood turbulence during rapid ventricular filling, and S_4 is due to blood turbulence during atrial systole (contraction of atria).

Chapter 4

Blood Pressure

The pressure which the blood exerts on the walls of the vessels is called *Blood Pressure*. Blood Pressure is normally recorded as systolic and diastolic pressure. The maximum pressure of blood in an artery is called *Systolic pressure* and is due to ventricular systole. The minimum pressure in an artery is called the *Diastolic pressure* which is due to ventricular diastole (relaxation of ventricles).

Pressure is generally much higher in arteries than in veins. When doctors talk about blood pressure they normally mean arterial pressure.

If blood pressure of a person is measured immediately after five miles of jogging or after he had delivered a speech, the reading would undoubtedly seem high, its natural. This is not a cause for alarm because its natural for blood pressure to rise and fall with changes in activity or emotional state. Its also normal for blood pressure to vary from person to person, even from one area of the body to another (The blood pressure is not of the same degree in all vessels. It is much more in those arteries which are near to the heart than in those which are further away from heart). But when blood pressure remains constantly high then it's an alarming sign. Like air in a tyre, too much air pressure can damage a tyre, similarly too much blood pressure can threaten healthy arteries. Constantly high blood pressure force heart to work for beyond its capacity. Besides injuring blood vessels, it can damage the brain, eyes, and kidneys. Hypertension is often called *'the silent killer'* because it rarely exhibits symptoms even as it inflicts serious damage on the body.

NORMAL VALUES OF BLOOD PRESSURE

The blood pressure of an individual is not a fixed entity. Normally it may vary considerably due to variety of factors, but it tends to assume the average for the age group. Normal blood pressure varies from individual to individual depending upon age, sex, dietetic habits and occupation. The systolic blood pressure normally fluctuates between 110 mmHg to 140 mmHg and diastolic pressure between 70 mmHg to 90 mmHg. Any increase in these figures is considered as high blood pressure and decrease is treated as low blood pressure.

The blood pressure is affected by age. In the young, blood pressure value is low while in the adult pressure value is generally 120/80 mmHg. Both the systolic and diastolic blood pressure rises gradually with age, but the rise is very gradual till about 40 years of age; from 40 years onward, the rise is particularly steep especially of systolic blood pressure. Normally at 70 years of age the blood pressure is 160/90 mmHg. In some areas of the world where modernism has not made sufficient inroads, the blood pressure is not influenced by age.

Efforts have been made to find out a rough and ready formula to calculate the normal blood pressure at a given age, but all these formulas have been put forward to work out the systolic pressure only and not the diastolic. Unfortunately no satisfactory formula has so far been found. It was once suggested the "age+100" formula, in which 100 is added to the age of individual. But "age+100" formula was discarded because the figures deduced for old age were often too high. Another formula was, in which 120 mmHg should be taken as normal systolic pressure at the age 20 and for every 2 years of age 1 mmHg should be added to 120. This has been found satisfactory but was discarded because it figured out very low blood pressure for the old age groups. Third formula of "age+90", in which 90 should be added to the age, to get normal systolic figure gives more correct values than any other formula.

Systolic pressure in young healthy adult varies from 100 to 130 mmHg and diastolic pressure varies from 60 to 80 mmHg. In women (before menopause) the pressure is usually slightly lower than in men.

CONTROL OF BLOOD PRESSURE

The mechanisms by which blood pressure is maintained are complicated. Blood pressure in the arteries must be controlled to ensure an adequate supply of blood and oxygen to the organs. If the arterial blood pressure is too low, the body tissues may not receive enough blood. If it is too high, it may damage blood vessels and organs.

Blood pressure is controlled mainly by the brain, autonomic nervous system, kidneys, some of the endocrine glands, arteries and the heart. The brain is the centre of blood pressure control in the body. It directs the various other organs of the body according to the body's demands and need. Rapid changes in blood pressure trigger compensatory responses from the nervous system within seconds. These automatic nervous responses do not involve the conscious part of the brain. Long-term changes are largely regulated by hormones. Hormonal responses work for over several hours.

Short-term Control of Blood Pressure

A sudden change in posture or heavy bleeding may cause a rapid change in blood pressure, to which the nervous system immediately responds. Nerve fibers that are part of the autonomic nervous system bring signals from all parts of the body to inform the brain of the status of the blood pressure, the volume of blood and the specialized need of all organs. This information is processed by the brain and decisions are automatically taken and messages are sent out via the outgoing nerves. These outgoing nerves end up in the organs (including their blood vessels), where the signal causes narrowing or opening of the vessels. An automatic response adjust the heart rate, volume of blood pumped and arterial diameter to restore normal pressure. These nerves function automatically without our knowledge.

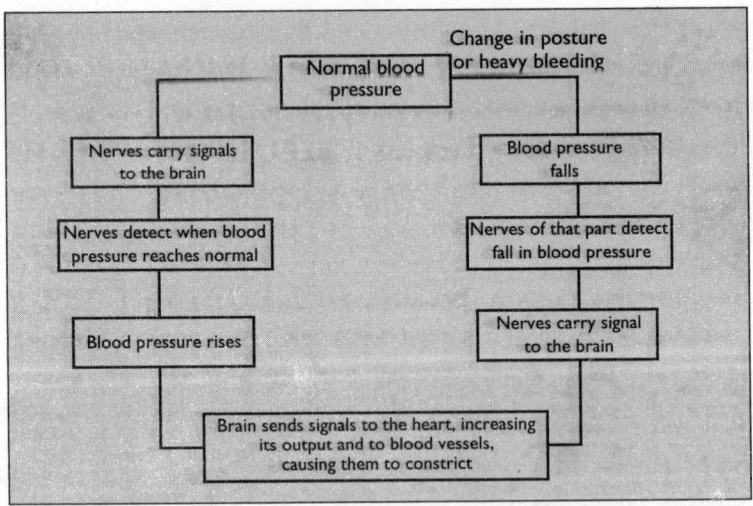

Flow chart showing response to falling blood pressure

Long Term Control of Blood Pressure

Blood pressure is controlled in the long term by action of hormones. Kidney is the regulator of fluids in the body. It responds to low blood pressure by secreting a hormone called *renin*, which raises the blood pressure. Renin from kidney stimulate the formation of *angiotensin*, which constrict arteries and raises blood pressure. Hormones from several organs also affect the blood pressure. The adrenal glands secretes several hormones that can control blood pressure, including *cortisone, adrenaline* and *aldosterone*. The thyroid gland, hypothalamus and ovaries also respond to high or low blood pressure by secreting hormones *thyroxine, ADH (antidiuretic hormone)* and *estrogen*, respectively. Although the hearts main function is to pump blood to the organs, it also secretes *Atrial Natriuretic Factor*, a hormone that can rid the body of excess salt and help keep the blood vessels properly dilated. All of these hormones are necessary for the body to function.

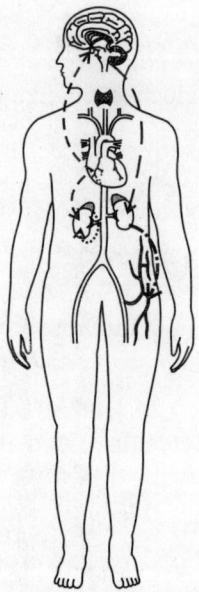

Fig. 7: Diagram showing long term control of blood pressure

The arteries themselves also contribute to blood pressure control. The muscles in the walls of the vessels can dilate to increase the blood supply to an organ, or contract to shunt blood away and distribute it where it is most wanted. For example, when we eat, blood is shifted to the bowel to help the digestion, and when we exercise, blood is shifted to the exercising muscles.

The functions of the kidney, hormones and arteries are not isolated. They are directed by the brain, but they also use their own systems according to their needs. For example if the blood supply of the kidney is blocked, the kidney can secrete renin without consulting brain.

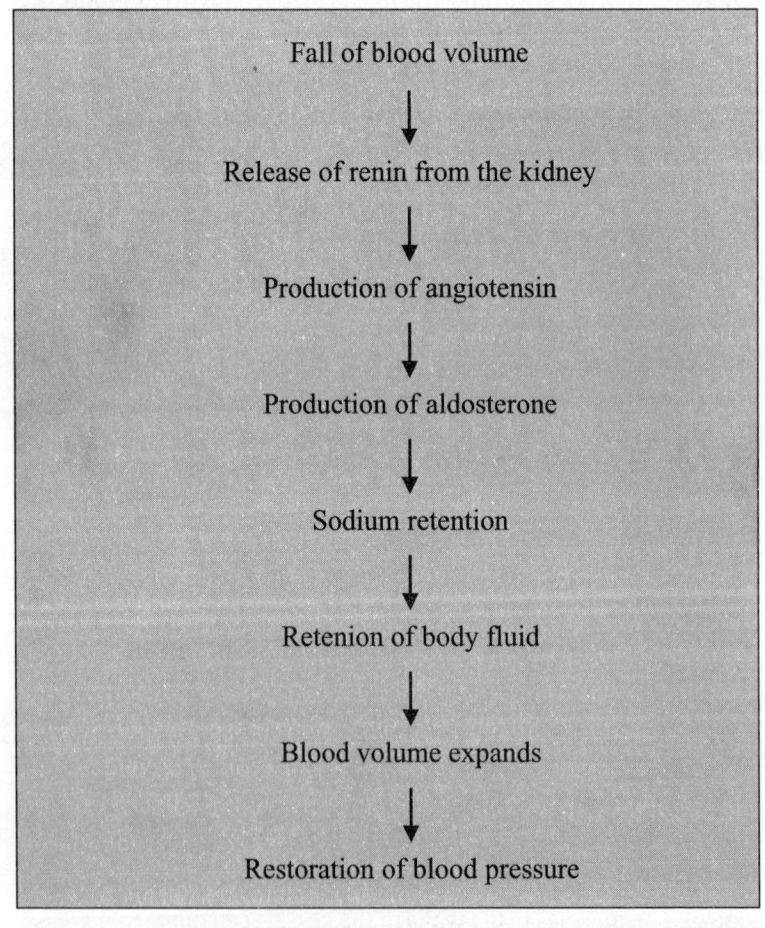

Fall of blood volume
↓
Release of renin from the kidney
↓
Production of angiotensin
↓
Production of aldosterone
↓
Sodium retention
↓
Retenion of body fluid
↓
Blood volume expands
↓
Restoration of blood pressure

Factors Controlling Blood Pressure

The pressure of blood is controlled by several variables:

1. Cardiac Output

Blood pressure varies directly with the cardiac output.

2. Blood Volume and Viscosity

Both viscosity and the volume of blood vary, depending mainly on salt intake, the size and shape of red blood cells, efficiency of kidney or level of alcohol in blood. Thus

If there is high volume of blood, suppression of ADH secretion causes diuresis resulting in reduction in blood volume.

3. Elasticity of Blood Vessels

If blood vessels loses their elasticity, systolic blood pressure rises but not the diastolic pressure.

4. Effect of Velocity

If the velocity of blood is very high blood pressure falls. The narrowing of blood vessels increases the velocity of blood. Thus, in aortic stenosis and in coarctation of aorta the blood pressure is very low.

5. Friction

When arterial walls get older, rougher and furred up with waxy plaques, made up of a mixture of cholesterol and blood clots, causes increased friction along arterial wall. This process raises blood pressure by increasing resistance to blood flow.

CONDITIONS AFFECTING BLOOD PRESSURE

1. Physiological Factors

- **Age**: Both the systolic and diastolic blood pressure rises gradually with age.

- **Sex**: After menopause (above 45 years), women have little higher blood pressure than males of similar age group. Before menopause women have lower blood pressure than males of similar age group.

- **Diurnal**: The blood pressure reading is the lowest when one awakes after sleep. During the day the blood pressure fluctuates but it tends to rise most in the evening. During sleep the blood pressure is the lowest. But in these fluctuation the systolic pressure is only affected.

- **Posture**: In the recumbent position blood pressure is the lowest, while when standing, the systolic pressure rises by about 10 mmHg and diastolic pressure also rises slightly.

- **Meals**: After meals the blood pressure is little higher. Generally systolic pressure raises not the diastolic. The bigger the meal, the greater is the rise.

- **Emotions**: Emotional states like rage, panic, depression, anger and excitement raises the blood pressure.

- **Exposure to Cold**: Exposure to cold causes rise of blood pressure.

- **Exercise**: In healthy individual exercise will cause rise of blood pressure. It causes rise of systolic pressure and fall of diastolic pressure.

2. Pathological Factors

- Blood pressure falls, sometimes alarmingly in cardiovascular shock and spinal shock.

- In great majority of cases of high blood pressure the etiology cannot be found (*Essential high blood pressure*). In a small percentage of cases the rise of blood pressure is due to some pathological condition or disease (*Secondary high blood pressure*).

3. Drug Induced

Many allopathic drugs produces alteration of blood pressure. Like after a powerful diuretic blood pressure falls. Drugs stimulating sympathetic nervous system raises blood pressure while relaxants of vascular smooth muscles reduces the blood pressure.

Chapter 5
High Blood Pressure

High blood pressure or hypertension means a persistently abnormal increase of blood pressure due to malfunction of one or several of the factors responsible for maintaining normal blood pressure. The word hypertension comes from translating the French phrase 'tension arterielle', this originally referred to tension in the walls of arteries.

Blood pressure varies naturally with activities, rising during exercise or stress and falling during rest. It also varies among individuals and gradually increases with age. In general, a person is considered to have high blood pressure or hypertension when his or her blood pressure is persistently higher than 140/90 mmHg, even at rest.

The higher the blood pressure, the greater the risk of complications such as heart attack, coronary artery disease and stroke. If a person having high blood pressure with several other risk factors for heart disease, such as high cholesterol, being a smoker or a family tendency to heart diseases, then treatment for high blood pressure is worth while. On the other hand, for some people with marginally raised blood pressure and no other risk factors for heart disease then treatment may be held back and such people should be kept under observation.

In the last few years, health education and screening programs have led to many more people being diagnosed with hypertension at an early stage before any complication occur. Early diagnosis, together with improved treatments, has substantially reduced the incidence of heart attacks and strokes due to high blood pressure.

AFFECTS OF HIGH BLOOD PRESSURE

If the blood pressure is higher than usual for many years, as in untreated hypertension, it can cause damage to the arteries of the body and to the organs they supply, especially the heart, brain and kidney.

Blood vessels are like rubber tube that carry blood to all over body. Arteries which carry blood out of the heart, have to withstand the great pressure with which the blood is pumped out. If the blood pressure is higher than normal over many years, the vessels get damaged. The lining of the arteries can become roughened and thickened and this eventually causes them to narrow and become less flexible. This condition is known as *arteriosclerosis*. If an artery becomes too narrow, blood cannot get through properly, and the part of the body that depends on that artery for its blood supply and oxygen content is starved of blood and oxygen that it carries. If an artery narrows there is an increased tendency to develop blood

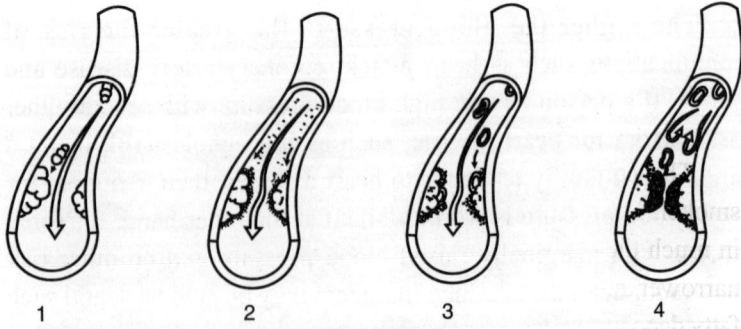

Fig. 8: Showing different stages of blockage in the arteries

clots, which may cause total blockage of the artery so that part of the body that it serves dies. If the brain or the heart is affected, the dead part is known as *infarct*. If the blood pressure elevation is mild, the increase in the rate of hardening of the artery is not usually great.

We must emphasize that most of the bad effects caused by high blood pressure can be prevented if the blood pressure is brought down to normal by treatment. It is also important to understand that factors such as smoking, high cholesterol and diabetes, can cause similar damage to the body and that these factors should also be controlled.

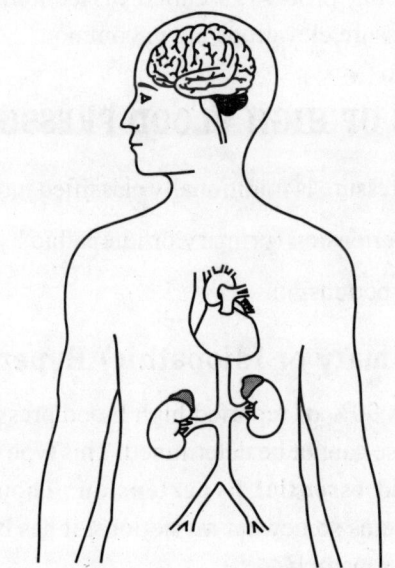

Fig. 9: Multi-dimensional effect of hypertension

The complications can be more severe if one is a cigarette smoker. The reason is that cigarette smoking damages blood vessels in much the same way as high blood pressure, making the artery narrower and its lining thick and rough. High cholesterol can cause fatty deposits, called atheroma to develop more rapidly than normal, which causes narrowing of the arteries. Diabetes can also contribute to narrowing of the arteries causing cardiovascular diseases. High glucose levels in the blood damage arteries in a similar way as high blood pressure.

If the blood pressure is severely elevated for a period of time, then the consequences come sooner and are usually much worse. Severely elevated pressure can sometimes cause the blood vessels to burst. When blood leaks out of a blood vessel it is called *hemorrhage*. Hemorrhage into the brain causes a serious, often fatal stroke. Severely elevated pressure can also cause the largest artery of the body, the aorta, to bulge known as *aneurysm*, and even burst. Bursting process is called *dissection*. Fortunately, serious blood pressure elevations are uncommon.

TYPES OF HIGH BLOOD PRESSURE

High blood pressure is traditionally classified into two groups:
- Essential hypertension (primary or idiopathic hypertension)
- Secondary hypertension.

Essential (Primary or Idiopathic) Hypertension

In as many as 90% of reported high blood pressure cases the under – lying cause cannot be determined. This type of high blood pressure is called **essential hypertension**. Though essential hypertension remains somewhat mysterious, it has been linked to certain risk factors, namely:
- Heredity
- More common in men
- Age & race
- Overweight
- High alcohol intake

Essential hypertension is also greatly influenced by life style. The link between salt and high blood pressure is especially compelling. The majority of all hypertensives are "salt sensitive", meaning that anything more than the minimal bodily need for salt is too much for them and leads to an increase in blood pressure. Example people living on the northern islands of Japan eat more salt per capita than anyone else in the world and exhibit the highest incidence of essential hypertension. By contrast, people who add no salt to their food show virtually no trace of essential hypertension.

Other factors associated with high blood pressure include:
- Diabetes
- Obesity
- Stress
- Chronic alcohol consumption
- Lack of physical activity
- Insufficient intake of potassium, magnesium & calcium

As more cases are discovered, even primary high blood pressure will eventually have to be recognized as a diverse group.

Secondary Hypertension

When a direct cause can be identified, the condition is described as **secondary hypertension**. Among the known causes of secondary hypertension, **kidney disease** ranks highest.

Secondary hypertension is also triggered by the following factors:
- Coarctation of aorta (a malformation of large artery that carries blood from the heart).
- By tumors of pituitary gland, adrenal glands or kidneys.
- By overproduction of some hormones known to raise blood pressure like adrenal hormones or thyroid hormones.

- By disorders involving compression of the brain or brainstem.
- Brain tumor or any cause of increased intracranial pressure.

These classical secondary cause altogether account for less than 1% of all treated cases of high blood pressure. Birth control pills (specifically those containing estrogen) and pregnancy can boost blood pressure, as can medication that constrict blood vessels.

Although the causes are diverse, the consequences of uncontrolled high blood pressure and the methods of controlling it are not. Whatever the cause of high blood pressure, the risk of stroke, heart failure, coronary heart disease and various other sorts of organ damage are increased. The aim of treatment for high blood pressure is usually to find drugs that work and are well tolerated.

High blood pressure is rare in childhood. However, when high blood pressure does occur in childhood, it may cause very serious and irreversible damage to the brain, eyes or kidney, if not treated. As it is so rare in childhood, the possibility is often forgotten and so the diagnosis may be made too late.

Malignant Hypertension

Patient who suffer organ damage as a result of high blood pressure are said to have malignant hypertension. If the blood pressure remain very high for weeks, months or years with a sustained diastolic pressure of at least 120 mmHg (usually much more) the walls of the smallest arteries (arterioles) begin to crumble. Blood then leaks out of them, interrupting the blood supply in whichever part of the body they happen to be. This usually begins in the kidney. The next site of damage is usually the retina (the back of the eye), causing retinal hemorrhage.

Malignant hypertension is a dangerous condition that develops rapidly and requires immediate medical attention. Despite the name it has nothing to do with cancer, but it is most serious form of high blood pressure. If it is not recognized and treated urgently, then irreversible damage to the kidneys, retina and brain is likely. Nowadays people with high blood pressure are picked up early by routine check-up, malignant hypertension is becoming rare.

White Coat Hypertension

It is not a type of high blood pressure that needs any treatment. Simply entering a hospital or a doctor's clinic can make some people so nervous that their blood pressure shoots up. If they are allowed some time to get over their initial fear, then their blood pressure returns to it normal level. The 'white coat' name comes from the fact that so many medical professionals (especially those in hospitals) wear white coats when they are working.

LOW BLOOD PRESSURE

Low blood pressure is not defined by a number, as is the case with high blood pressure; rather only the presence of symptoms indicates there is a problem. While most of the people in any typical large group of adults will have normal blood pressure, there will be few who have high blood pressure and few who have low blood pressure.

There is consistent evidence that mature adults whose systolic pressure is about 95–105 mmHg (very low) are more likely to feel less energetic, easily tired or mildly depressed than people with higher pressure, although they are likely to live longer. The only symptom of low blood pressure is **fainting**. If blood pressure in neck arteries is not high enough to supply enough oxygen and glucose to support the full functions of brain cells, then a person can feel dizzy. If this continues or becomes more severe, he/she can faint. This is more likely to occur when he/she stands up. This certainly can be nuisance and can sometimes have serious consequences, for example, if the person falls and breaks his bone. In teenagers (particularly girls) this happens easily and often, because their blood pressure is generally very low (systolic pressure under 100 mmHg is common) and often less stable than in mature adults. The same thing will happen if blood pressure is brought down too low by over treatment. Low blood pressure may lead to symptom such as fatigue.

Fortunately, the complications of low blood pressure are not as severe as those of high blood pressure.

■

Chapter 6

Causes

In 95 percent of cases of high blood pressure there is no specific underlying cause and this condition is known as primary or essential hypertension. However, both lifestyle and genetic factors may contribute. There are many features which are commonly associated with high blood pressure–that is, they occur more often in people with high blood pressure than in people with low blood pressure. It is not always easy to test, whether these associations are also causes or simply coincidences.

The condition is most common in aged and elderly people because the arteries become more rigid with age. Blood pressure tends to increase with age, but this is partly because of changes in lifestyle. Many people put on weight and get less active as they get older and both these factors may contribute to the development of high blood pressure. More importantly, the rise in blood pressure with age is greater in people who eat a lot of salty foods.

The tension in hypertension refers to the tension in the artery walls and not to the sought of tension people generally talk about, stress and worry. Stress is one possible cause of otherwise unexplained high blood pressure, but it is not the only cause, and may not even be a common cause. A stressful lifestyle may aggravate the condition. High blood pressure therefore occurs most often in developed countries. It has been found out that lots of nervous people have normal or even low blood pressures, and lots of easy going phlegmatic people have dangerously high blood pressures. Clearly there are many other good reasons for avoiding or eliminating social and psychological stresses, regardless of any possible effect on blood pressure.

Apart from inheritance, there is good evidence that there are four factors which are true and independent causes of high blood pressure. These factors are:

- Overweight
- High sodium (salt) intake
- Low potassium intake
- High alcohol intake

Blood pressure always varies throughout the day and is usually higher during exercise as the heart needs to pump blood faster, although people who exercise regularly will tend to have lower blood pressure than non-active people. Blood pressure is lower while sleeping or resting. But a person will not be diagnosed as hypertensive on the basis of a one-off reading. At least two-high (i.e. over 160/90 mmHg) readings on three separate occasions, over at least two months is necessary to diagnose a person '*hypertensive*'.

In pregnant women, high blood pressure can lead to the development of the potentially life-threatening conditions. The elevated blood pressure usually returns to normal after the delivery.

Though essential hypertension remains somewhat mysterious, it has been linked to certain risk factors. In only about one to two of 100 cases a treatable cause can be found.

The most common easily treated causes of elevated blood pressure are:

1. Heredity

An individual's blood pressure level depends on the interplay of genetic or inherited factors and influences of the persons lifestyle. It is known that heredity plays a large part in developing high blood pressure. At least half of the cases of high blood pressure can be predicted from knowledge of blood pressure in parents, brothers and sisters. High blood pressure clearly runs in families, and this holds true even after allowances have been made for the fact that families tend to share the same lifestyle and diet.

Excellent research has been conducted among twins who were brought up separately or together and also among adopted children compared with non-adopted children, to identify how much of the similarity in blood pressure within families is the result of inheritance compared with the proportion resulting from similarities in lifestyle. Roughly about half of all the variations in blood pressure is the result of genetic factors.

However, it is yet not clear exactly how it is inherited. Though it is known that some of the characteristics (like the color of eyes) and some rare diseases can be caused by inheriting a single gene but high blood pressure is hardly ever inherited in this simple way. It is more important to realize that there may be a possibility of developing high blood pressure, when family history of high blood pressure is present and that person should therefore be sensible about what he eats and drinks, the amount of exercise he takes and should not smoke.

Blood pressure depends on interaction between different inherited factors, many of which operated if certain environmental factors exist. The most important of these conditions are:

- Premature babies tends to develop high blood pressure in middle age
- Being considerably overweight in adolescence and as a young adult

- Alcohol intake particularly in younger people

As to preventing it, there is as yet no evidence that this can be done but there are two likely possibilities. One is to reduce sodium intake, the other is to keep weight within normal levels for age and height.

2. Salt Intake

Things that a person eats and drinks can affect his/her blood pressure. Salt intake has a direct effect on blood pressure. Reducing salt intake helps to reduce blood pressure.

A high salt intake over many years probably raises blood pressure by raising the sodium content of the smooth muscle cells of the walls of the arterioles. The high sodium content appear to facilitate the entry of calcium into the cells, this in turn causes them to contract and narrows the internal diameter of the arteriole. There is some evidence that people with an inherited tendency to develop hypertension have a reduced capacity to remove salt from their bodies. It is certainly true, that there are variations in the way individual bodies handle salt and some people are more sensitive to it than others. It is also evident that older people are more salt-sensitive.

The Japanese, Polish and Portuguese have high salt intake and a high frequency of raised blood pressure and strokes. If children could be persuaded to consume less salt then we might prevent the development of hypertension.

3. Age and Sex

High blood pressure is more likely to affect men than women. At or after the menopause women are prone to suffer from high blood pressure.

Blood pressure usually rises with age and is mostly found in people after the age of forty but young people also suffer from

Causes

high blood pressure. The high blood pressure in younger adults are generally secondary to other disorders (usually affecting the kidney or the adrenal glands). Doctors should refer everyone aged under 40 and found to have high blood pressure for special investigations to see if it has been caused by any such disorders.

Many cases are seen even below the age of twenty, as also in children of about 10 years of age. The cause of high blood pressure may not be same in all these people. High blood pressure in children is almost always due to a chronic inflammation of the kidneys.

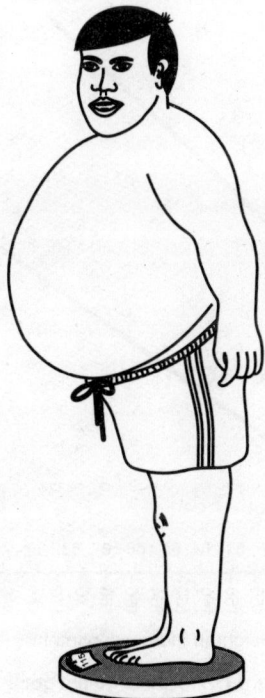

Fig. 10: Obesity in relation to hypertension

4. Over Weight (Obesity)

More cases of high blood pressure are found in the over-weight and obese individuals than in thin and under-weight people. This is partly because obese people have to work harder to burn up the excess calories they consume, partly because they tend to eat more salt than normal.

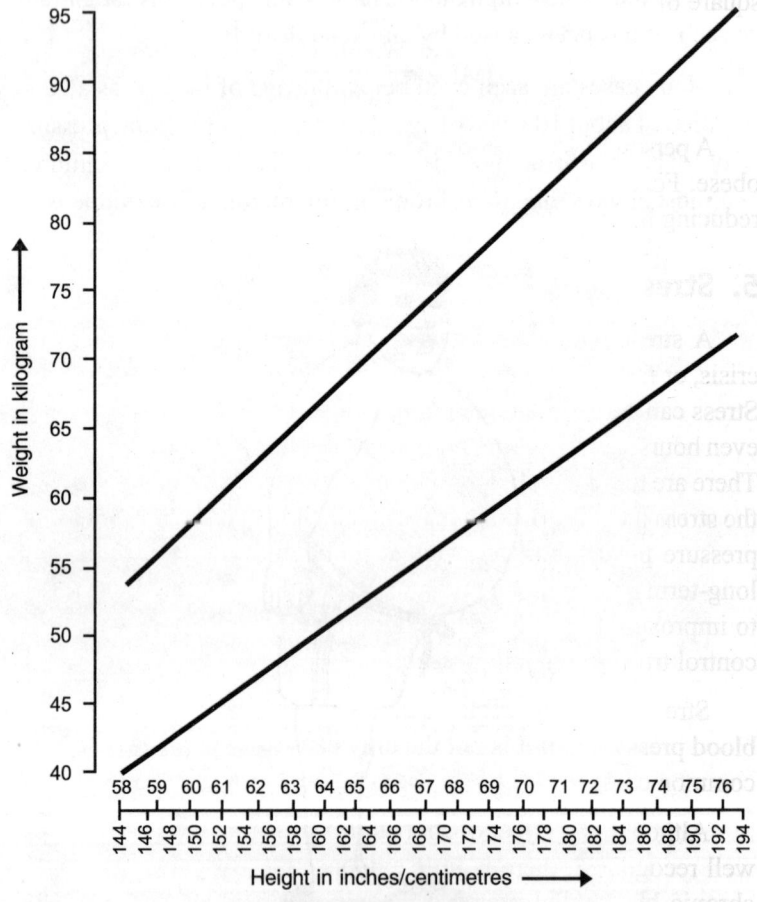

Fig. 11: Height & weight graph

The relationship between body weight and blood pressure is more complex than was originally thought, and it may also be related to important effect of certain hormones, as well as to the body's capacity to handle salt. It is not possible to say whether you are over-weight just on the basis of how much you actually weigh because tall people usually weigh more than short people, so instead doctors usually work out on body mass index (BMI). BMI is calculated by taking weight in kilograms and dividing it by the square of your height in meters.

$$BMI = \frac{Weight\ (Kg)}{[Height(m)]^2}$$

A person who has a body mass index of 30 or more is considered obese. For obese person losing weight is a very effective way of reducing blood pressure.

5. Stress

A stressful situation such as a problem at work, a financial crisis, or family trouble can raise your blood pressure temporarily. Stress can cause a rapid rise in blood pressure, lasting minutes or even hours. Such rises are normal and occur in stressed individuals. There are temporary peaks in blood pressure—they go away when the stress that causes them is removed. Stress can raise your blood pressure in the short term but it probably does not account for long-term rises in blood pressure. Relaxation techniques may help to improve the quality of life, but probably will not be enough to control true high blood pressure.

Stress is one possible cause of otherwise unexplained high blood pressure, but it is not the only cause and may not even be a common cause.

Although the effect of short-term stress on blood pressure are well recognized, there is little evidence that chronic stress cause chronic high blood pressure. People who suffer from continual anxiety or worry for many years, tend to become chronic hypertensive. A continued and sustained rise of blood pressure for a long stretch of time, caused by such mental factors may ultimately become a permanent disease.

Reliable studies have shown no relationship between level of stress, as assessed by detail and accurate questioning, and blood pressure. People with very stressful jobs do not have more high blood pressure or heart disease than people with less stressful jobs. Instead its known that lots of very nervous people have normal or even low blood pressure and lot of easy-going phlegmatic people have dangerously high blood pressure. There is some evidence that people who have less control over their day-to-day life at work have higher blood pressure than people who can influence their working life more effectively.

6. Alcohol Intake

There is no evidence to support, that moderate use of alcohol has any causative effect on blood pressure. But excessive amount of alcohol may be a contributory factor, either by its poisonous effect or by its capacity to make the drinker obese. The more alcohol you drink the higher your blood pressure, although it is not understood why? Interestingly, teetotallers tend to have slightly higher blood pressure than moderate drinkers, heavy drinkers are very likely to have raised blood pressure and also have a strong tendency to develop strokes. When such people stop drinking their

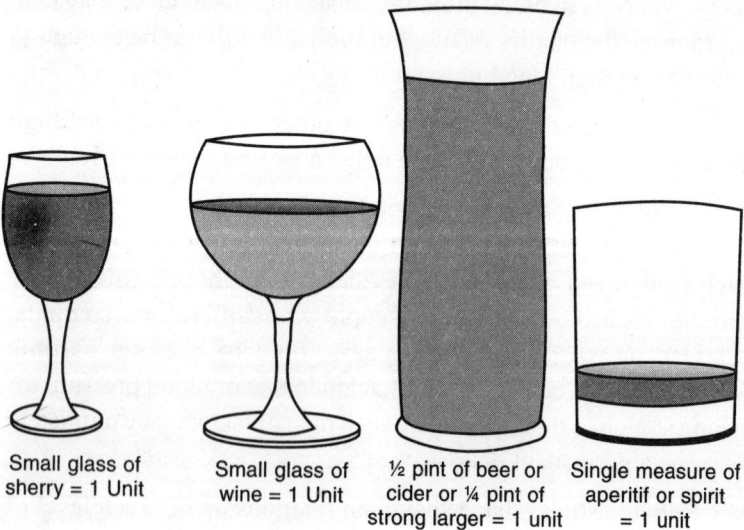

Fig. 12: Units of alcohol

blood pressure comes down. Alcohol increases fat in the body and the resulting obesity further aggravates the problem.

Doctors recommend that men should drink no more than 21 units of alcohol per week (equivalent to 10½ pint of beer or 21 small glasses of wine) and women should drink no more than 14 units per week (equivalent to 7 pints of beer or 14 small glasses of wine). These should be spread over the week, not drunk all at once. A unit of alcohol is equivalent to approximately 8–10 grams of pure alcohol.

7. Medicines

Some drugs, both prescribed and non-prescribed (bought over the counter), increases blood pressure. The most commonly used drugs that can elevate blood pressure are **birth control pills** and other hormone pills that contain estrogen. All corticosteroid hormones and adrenocorticotrophic hormones and other hormones, if given in high dosage, raises blood pressure by causing sodium and water retention and thus increases the volume of blood in the body. Large doses of steroid tablets or injections should never be used other than for serious, usually life-threatening disease, which will usually be under the care of doctors.

Medicines for cold, hay fever, chronic catarrh or allergy that contain decongestants, for shrinking up of the nasal air passages, can constrict the blood vessels and raise blood pressure. So, these should not be used unnecessarily and in high dosages. Traditional remedies such as menthol or eucalyptus are safer and just as effective.

NSAIDs (Non steroidal anti-inflammatory drugs) like ibuprofen, which are commonly used for joint-pains, can also cause a substantial rise in blood pressure in most people. Because of this effect, it is important that you remind your doctor or pharmacist that you have high BP if you ever need painkillers.

8. Exercise

Vigorous forms of exercise such as running certainly causes

huge but brief rise in blood pressure. There is no evidence to support the idea that physical stresses such as exercise are a cause of high blood pressure. On the contrary regular exercise tends to keep one healthier with lower blood pressure compared to people who do not take exercise. There is good evidence that dynamic exercise such as cycling, running or swimming can reduce blood pressure as well as other risk factors for coronary disease (such as blood cholesterol and fibrinogen). This is partly because people who exercise are more likely to eat healthy foods, not smoke and not drink excessive alcohol, although exercise seems to have a direct effect on lowering blood pressures. One should aim to take regular, moderate amounts of exercise rather than going in for very vigorous bouts every now and then.

Static exercise as weight training, push-ups and other body-building exercise, can raise blood pressure substantially for brief period and can be dangerous in people who already have high blood pressure.

9. Tobacco

Regular and frequent consumption of tobacco (in the form of chewing, snuffing and smoking) gives rise to high blood pressure.

10. Calcium and Potassium

There is quite good evidence that people who have a low-potassium diet have higher blood pressure, whereas those who eat a lot of fruit and vegetables have lower blood pressure and few incidence of stroke. Having diet that contain potassium—such as fruits and vegetables—is good for keeping blood pressure low.

Potassium does seem to be beneficial in its own right. This makes sense because it is known that cells respond to high potassium by getting rid of sodium (salt).

There has been some research to suggest that a diet high in calcium may be protective against high blood pressure.

■

Chapter 7

Symptoms

The vast majority of people with high blood pressure have no symptoms. The fact that high blood pressure cause no symptoms means that it is often not diagnosed for many years, by which time the person has subtle evidence of damage to his or her heart, brain or kidneys. Symptoms do not appear as soon as the pressure tends to rise. At a later stage they may go to their doctor because they have started to feel sick. Often patients have no complaints, before a physician tells them about their heightened blood pressure. By itself before it has caused organ damage, high blood pressure causes no symptoms at all. In fact there is some evidence that people with uncomplicated high blood pressure may feel slightly better, more alert and energetic, than people with lower blood pressure.

When, however, the pressure reaches the limit of the patients tolerance, symptoms begin to appear. If symptoms do occur they may include:

- Headache
- Chest pain or tightness
- Breathless on exertion
- Palpitation

- Giddiness
- Sleep disturbances
- Nosebleeds
- Sub-conjunctival hemorrhage and impairment of vision
- Stroke
- Numbness and tingling
- Nervousness and irritability
- Excessive perspiration
- Muscle cramps
- Weakness
- Frequent urination
- Swelling under the eyes in the morning

Headache is one of the most common symptom of high blood pressure. There are several other causes of headache. Therefore one should be very careful about jumping to the conclusion. Nearly everyone gets ordinary headaches at some time or the other, which can be caused by anxiety, tension, mental strain, sleepless nights, indigestion or minor viral infections. Such headaches are equally common in people with high blood pressure, but a careful doctor will always check blood pressure first. Some of these headaches can be a warning of early damage to arteries of the brain or retina, requiring urgent control of blood pressure to prevent serious complications.

Breathlessness in people with high blood pressure is usually as a result of being overweight. However, if blood pressure has risen out of control then breathlessness may be the main symptom of heart ailments. When the heart is embarrassed by the increased load, breathlessness on slight exertion and cough appear.

Occasionally the patient feels giddy. There may be several other causes for this giddiness, namely cervical spondylitis, anemia, sleeplessness, disturbances in the internal ear and so on. Palpitation (feeling or hearing your own heart beat), headaches and over breathing are symptoms of anxiety are common in people. People may get palpitation for the first time after they have been told that they have high blood pressure. But it is due to fear and not due to high blood pressure. Some time palpitation is due to secondary high blood pressure, possibly caused by a tumor or an adrenal gland disorder.

Bleeding in and from different parts of the body is also the effect of hypertension. The risk of bleeding from arteries into the brain or into the retina (the back of the eye) is increased by high blood pressure, particularly in people over 50. Bleeding from nose and gums is common, and is deemed beneficial—since such bleeding may be considered as a safety-valve action. Nose bleeding and sub-conjunctival bleeding happen more often in people with high blood pressure, although both are very common in people with normal blood pressure. Sub-conjunctival bleeding is simply a small amount of bleeding in the white of the eye, it is completely harmless. Rapid failure of vision, or even sudden blindness occur due to retinal bleeding.

Bleeding in the brain is a very serious condition which kills the patient out-right or leaves him with paralysis. Due to high blood pressure the arteries supplying blood to the brain might burst as a result of which a part of the brain might get damaged. The damaged part of the brain causes paralysis or loss of functions of a particular part of the body. The patient generally gets such attack during day when he is active. This is generally called a **stroke**. The patient may become unconscious as a result of this stroke. Only occasionally a complete or almost complete recovery is seen.

Commonly, symptoms of the nervous system appear first, which are noticed by the patient-himself or by his relatives. Nervousness, irritability, inability to concentrate sleeplessness, headache and giddiness are some of the common initial symptoms.

Malfunctioning of the kidneys is one of the causative factors of high blood pressure and it inturns impairs the proper working of the kidneys. With the deterioration of the function of the kidneys the patient will need to get up several times for passing urine and puffiness under the eyes are noticed. The patient is thirsty and easily tired.

When the heart functions are affected by high blood pressure, increase load on heart causes breathlessness on slight exertion. Soon after, edema of ankles start, which is particularly marked in the evening after the days work. Pericardial distress, excessive perspiration and even anginal pain may be experienced. It may cause heart failure.

Severe high blood pressure in childhood usually shows up first as headaches but occasionally as fits or as impaired vision. A child with any of these symptoms, whether having them repeatedly or for the first time, should be taken to the doctor.

Heavy periods and menopausal symptoms such as palpitation, night sweats and hot flushes all commonly occur in women with high blood pressure.

These all are serious problems that is why one should never wait until they feel ill before getting their blood pressure checked. The current opinion is that every one over the age of 30 should have a routine blood pressure check. If the reading is normal then no action is required. Some people with borderline pressures may need to be checked more often.

Chapter 8

Diagnosis and Investigations

Simply measuring the blood pressure is by far the most important routine test for diagnosis of high blood pressure. It is important to make sure that enough reliable measurements have been made to allow an average blood pressure value to be calculated accurately and thus to assess how big the problem is! Except in extreme emergencies at least three readings on separate days are necessary.

SPHYGMOMANOMETER

The sphygmomanometer is the most common device used to measure blood pressure. Sphygmomanometer is simply the technical term for an instrument used to measure blood pressure. These instruments could equally be called as blood pressure monitors. The blood pressure measurements are expressed in millimeters of mercury.

The sphygmomanometer a device for measuring pressure connected to an inflatable cuff which is wrapped around upper arm. The three different types of the pressure measuring device are mercury aneroid and electronic.

Mercury Sphygmomanometer

This is the type of sphygmomanometer still used by most

doctors. It consists of an inflatable cuff attached to a long hollow glass tube with a mercury reservoir at its base. Blood pressure pushes the mercury up the tube and the level it reaches can then be read off on the scale.

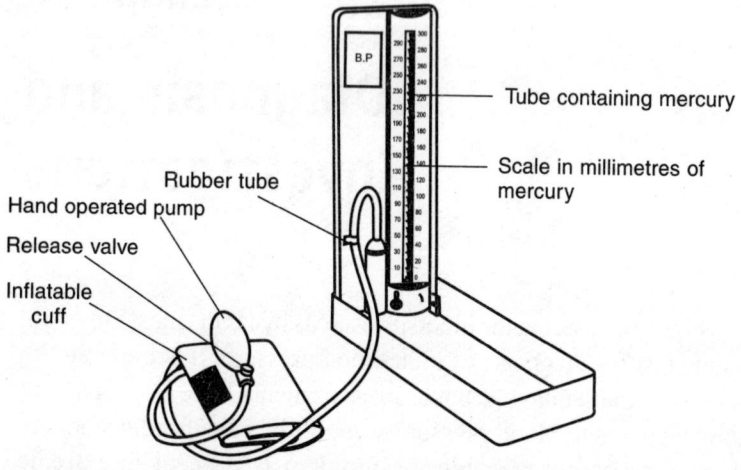

Fig. 13: Mercury sphygmomanometer

Aneroid Sphygmomanometer

This balances your blood pressure against pressure in a thin metal capsule containing air. Blood pressure is indicated by the position of a needle on a circular dial.

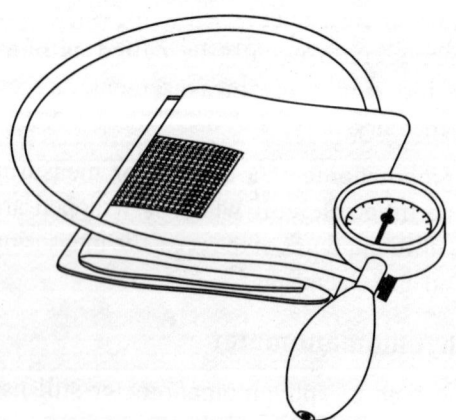

Fig. 14: Aneroid sphygmomanometer

Electronic Sphygmomanometer

In electronic sphygmomanometer, the pressure measuring device has a sensor in a cuff. This may be a microphone, which recognizes the appearance and disappearance of regular tapping sound, or a transducer which recognize a pulse wave. All one needs to do is to place the cuff around the arm and then press a button. One can take as many readings as necessary. Microprocessors convert the information received by the sensor into blood pressure reading, which is shown on machines display screen. If one does buy electronic sphygmomanometer, he/she can take it into the hospital or clinic so that doctor can quickly check the accuracy of the equipment against the mercury sphygmomanometer 'gold standard.'

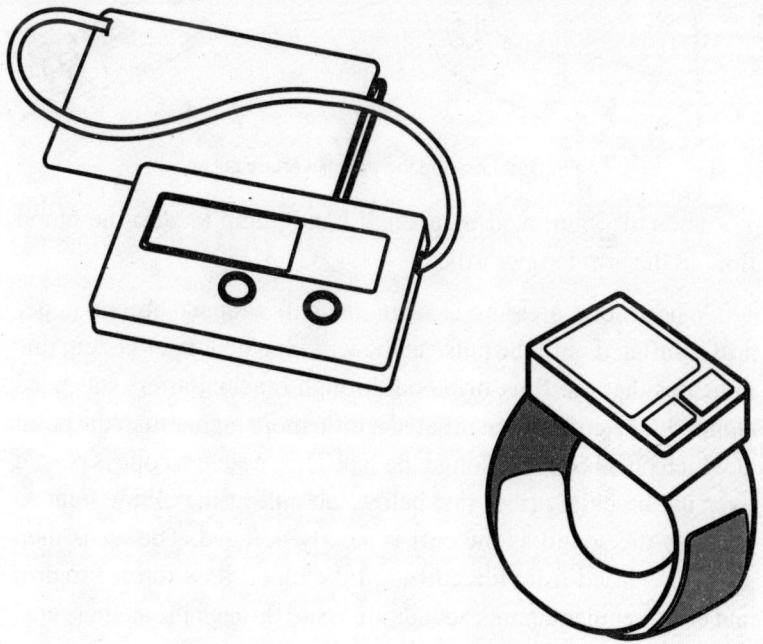

Fig. 15: Electronic sphygmomanometer

MEASURING BLOOD PRESSURE

The measurement of blood pressure is simple, quick and virtually painless. A proper sized cuff is placed around the upper arm. To hear the sounds of the heart pumping blood through the main artery in the arm, a stethoscope is placed in the crook of your elbow. The pressure required first to start and then to stop the sound is used as the measure of blood pressure.

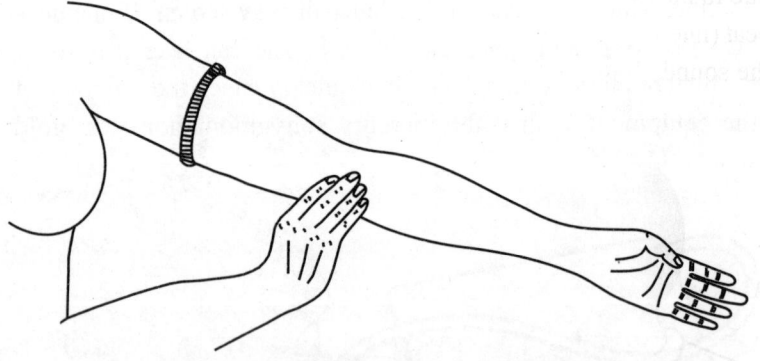

Fig. 16: Locating the brachial artery pulse

The cuff is inflated by a small hand pump to stop the blood flow in the arm temporarily.

When blood pressure is taken, the cuff wrapped around upper arm is inflated until the pulse in the wrist can no longer be felt; this indicates that the flow of blood through brachial artery has been stopped. The cuff is then inflated a little more higher than the point at which pulse could no longer be felt. Then a stethoscope is placed over the brachial artery just below the cuff at the elbow joint to listen to the sound as the cuff is slowly deflated. The air is then slowly released from the cuff until the blood flow returns to arm and clear, regular tapping sounds are heard through the stethoscope.

The level of pressure at which the first sound is heard corresponds to the systolic blood pressure and the figure shown on the sphygmomanometer scale recorded. The pressure in the cuff is then released further. The tapping sound disappears, it indicates that the blood is once again flowing smoothly through brachial artery. The level of pressure at which the sounds disappear, corresponds to the diastolic pressure and the figure on the sphygmomanometer scale is recorded. The pressure applied in the arm cuff is measured in millimeters of mercury (mmHg). The tapping sounds between the systolic and diastolic pressures are due to the blood in the artery flows past for only part of each heart beat (intermittent-flow), this turbulence of blood in the artery causes the sound.

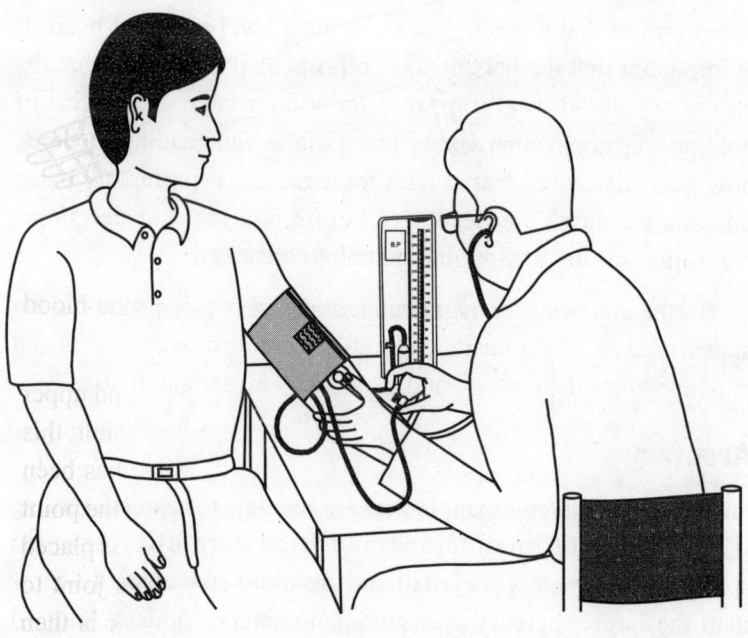

Fig. 17: A Doctor measuring blood pressures using a sphygmomanometer

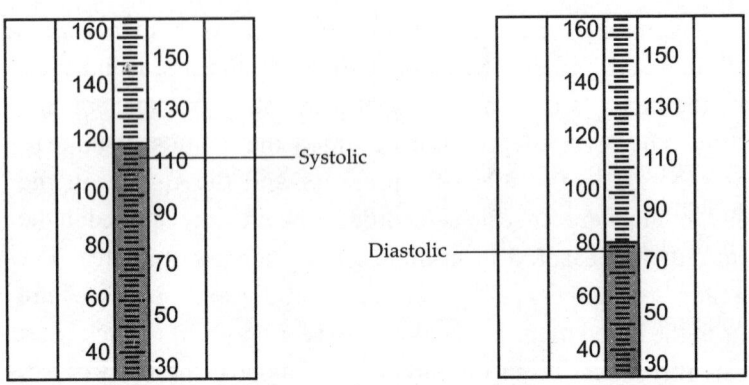

Fig. 18: Blood pressure reading – In this case is 120/80 mmHg

Usually, one is asked to sit down and the cuff is applied to upper arm so that it is roughly at the same level as that of heart. It is important that the person is as relaxed as possible and that the arm is supported by resting the elbow on a table—the effort of holding it up could otherwise produce a false high reading. Doctors, now generally agree that at least three readings (preferably made on separate days) are necessary before any real big decisions, regarding starting or stopping treatment are taken.

In the *electronic sphygmomanometer*, a sensor perceives the appearance and disappearance of pulse sounds or movements and machine notes the systolic and diastolic pressure automatically.

Accuracy

Mercury sphygmomanometers are accurate to nearest 2 mmHg if they are well maintained and used carefully. Aneroid sphygmomanometers are small and are more convenient to carry than the larger mercury sphygmomanometers. Modern Aneroid sphygmomanometers developed in the past few years are accurate and reliable, older instruments are not.

Electronic sphygmomanometers do not use mercury column to measure the pressure, they still report the blood pressure in millimeters of mercury, so that the reading obtained are comparable to those from the mercury 'good standard' system. They are also easy to use, particularly by people measuring their own blood pressure at home. But, unlike the traditional mercury instrument if may not be obvious it anything goes wrong with electronic sphygmomanometer, and the user may go on recording systematically incorrect and misleading readings. It makes little difference which type of equipment is being used when blood pressure is being taken because the procedure involved is much the same.

Blood pressure measurements need to be made carefully and by people who have been trained in how to take them. Apart from carelessness, the main source of human error come from using a cuff that is too small (on people with thick arms) or deflating the cuff too fast. If arm circumference is more than 35 cm, the cuff will not cut off the circulation sufficiently when inflated, so the reading may be overestimate of true blood pressure.

In order to get an accurate reading, the pressure in the cuff must be deflated at roughly 2 mmHg per second. If it is deflated faster than this, then blood pressure will be systematically underestimated, by an amount proportional to the speed of deflation. The faster the deflation the less accurate the reading.

Measurements on people with exceptionally thin arms underestimate blood pressure by 5–10 mmHg, however, carefully they are performed. It is probably the reason why research studies generally show that high blood pressure in very thin people appears to carry greater risks than the same levels of blood pressure in fat people.

Obviously these problems are not insurmountable—they can all be easily avoided by being careful and paying attention to detail.

Apart from recent exertion, pain, anger, embarrassment, fear and so on, the other important causes of misleading blood pressure reading are, some kind of meditation and a full bladder.

A stretched bladder causes a huge rise in blood pressure transiently i.e. people whose blood pressure is normally around 130/70 mmHg may easily rise to 200/120 mmHg in this way. This can happen easily anywhere if someone does not passes urine for a long time. It can also happen to men with prostate enlargement. Once a stretched bladder is emptied, blood pressure falls quickly to its usual value. Several commonly used drugs tend to raise blood pressure.

Children in general, right up to and probably during adolescence, tend to have even more variable blood pressure than adults, with huge differences between reading even when these seem to have been made in exactly the same circumstances. There are big problems about matching the measuring device to the size of a child arm. For at least the first year of child, systolic blood pressure can be measured only with either an ultrasound or an infrasound device, using only a very small cuff, with a specially trained observer taking the measurements. Diastolic blood pressure cannot be measured at all. Ultrasound machines are necessary up to about 8 years of age, with a range of cuff sizes. From about 10 years on, ordinary adult sphygmomanometers can be used but with small-sized cult. Many separate readings are necessary to define even a rough average pressure in a child.

Measuring Blood Pressure at Home

Home measurements have the great advantage that they can be made when the person is relaxed, and that he can make them as often as he like. There are several ways for measuring blood pressure away from hospital or clinics and this can be done by:

- A relative can be shown how to measure blood pressure and this may provide useful information
- A person may take his blood pressure with the help of electronic automatic blood pressure machines, although many of these are not very accurate. A typical blood pressure cuff is placed

around the arm and a button has to be pressed. One can take as many readings as necessary.

- Blood pressure can also be measured with a conventional mercury sphygmomanometer and a stethoscope at home. All people doing self-monitoring should have proper training in the method and need to have their machine checked periodically for accuracy. First you will need to support your measurement arm at about the same level as your heart (the level of the nipple in men). This usually means supporting your arm on a table and you may need a small cushion or book under your arm to ensure that it is at the right height. Make sure that the sphygmomanometer is so placed that you can see the scale easily. Wrap the inflatable cuff neatly round your upper arm. Fit the earpieces of the stethoscope into both your ears. Find your brachial artery pulse and put the diaphragm of the stethoscope over it. If you tuck half the diaphragm under the cult, it will leave your right hand free to operate the bulb that inflate the cuff.

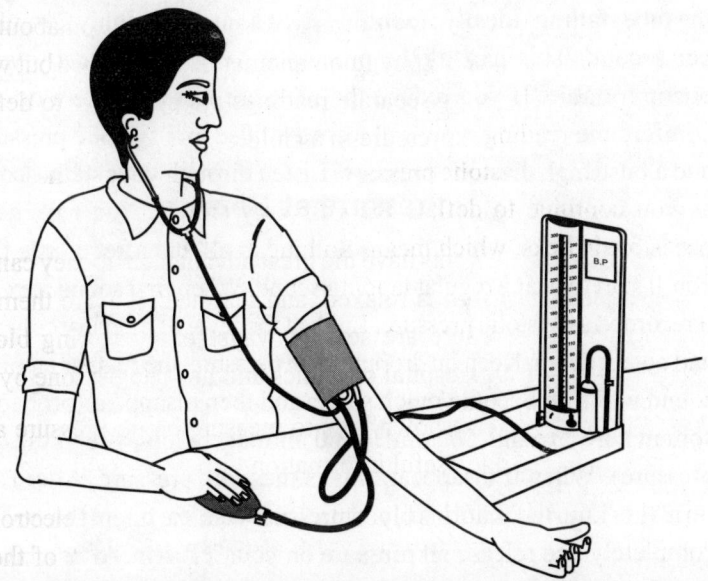

Fig. 19: Measuring your own blood pressure with a mercury sphygmomanometer

Turn your left hand palm upward. Take the inflating bulb in your right hand. With your left hand, tighten up the knurled screw clockwise until the valve is closed. By repeatedly squeezing the bulb with the valve closed, pump up the pressure on the glass column, now and then checking your pulse in your left wrist. The reason you have to keep checking the pulse is that when it disappears, it's a signal that you've pushed the pressure in the cuff above systolic pressure. As blood pressure varies so much, different people need to start measuring it from different levels. Of course, we could suggest that everyone should start from 250 mmHg or more, higher than expected systolic pressure but this would inflict a lot of unnecessary pain on the people whose systolic pressure lies 150 mmHg or lower than this—so you tailor the procedure to 20 mmHg or so above your own systolic pressure. For example your wrist pulse disappear at around 160 mmHg, keep on squeezing the bulb another 20 mmHg or so, then stop.

Now, very slowly and cautiously, start turning the knurled nut anticlockwise until you see the top of the column of mercury, in the tube, falling. Ideally it should fall at a rate of roughly 2 mmHg per second. This part of the process is very slow, usually very uncomfortable. If you reduce the pressure fast to make a quick, comfortable reading, you will record a false low systolic pressure and a false high diastolic pressure. Listen through your stethoscope as you continue to deflate the cuff very slowly. You may hear occasional clicks, which means nothing at all, but after a little fall you'll start to hear a regular tapping sound. When first sound appear, it recorded as systolic pressure. Look at the level of mercury column and note it down. Keep on dropping the pressure, the regular tapping sound will first become much softer and then disappear (probably somewhere around 50 mmHg–60 mmHg below your systolic pressure). When it disappear, this is diastolic pressure. After that turn the knurled knob fully anticlockwise to open the valve completely and release all pressure on your left arm. After a bit of practice you'll find you can do this easily and more quickly.

Diagnosis and Investigations

You will actually be hearing the sound of the blood flowing through your brachial artery. When the cuff is inflated enough to stop the blood flowing, there is no sound. As soon as the pressure from the cuff falls below this peak pressure, blood starts to flow. At first, at or below systolic pressure but above diastolic pressure, it flows continuously. As pressure reduces in the cuff you can hear these spurts of blood (with stethoscope), first as a tapping sound, later as a longer, softer whoosing sound and finally the sound disappear. The first regular tapping sound is your systolic pressure. After reducing pressure in the cuff eventually sound disappear, that's your diastolic pressure.

Ambulatory Blood Pressure Monitoring

Portable automatic blood pressure measuring device can record blood pressure many times throughout the day (24-hour). These

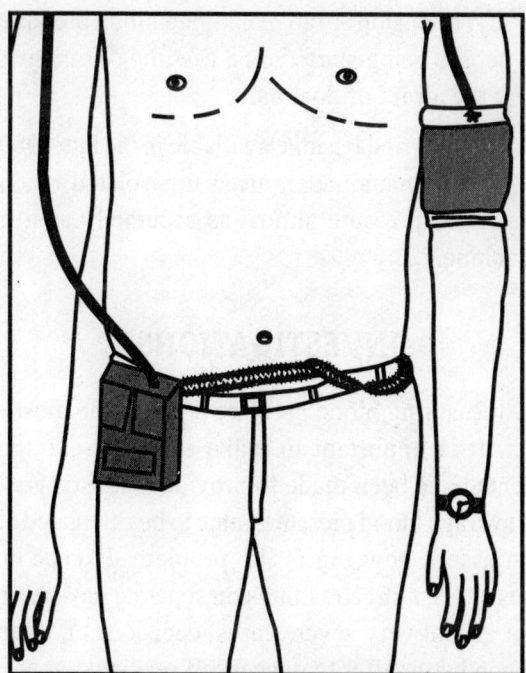

Fig. 20: An automatic 24 hours ambulatory monitor to record a person's blood pressure

24-hour ambulatory blood pressure monitor (ABPM) is reliable and accurate and can be programmed to measure the blood pressure every half hour or so over 24 hours.

A typical blood pressure cuff is worn, and a small pump inflates and deflates the cuff automatically. These machines are no longer than a paperback book and are worn on the belt or a shoulder strap. They are reasonably comfortable to wear and these machines at night does not often cause any sleep disturbance. Information is stored in the units memory and later transferred to a computer for printout.

With these machines, an average blood pressure can be determined during many different activities. They do not interfere in ordinary activities of a more sedentary kind, but heavy work is impossible. Ambulatory blood pressure monitoring is still mainly a research tool. But it is an accurate method of sorting out 'white coat' hypertension' from real higher blood pressure and thus preventing people being started on a lifetime of treatment merely because they are afraid of doctors.

These machines first became available in the late 1980s. Unlike electronic sphygmomanometers used for isolated readings, they do measure blood pressure almost as accurately as a traditional mercury machine.

INVESTIGATIONS

Simply measuring blood pressure is by far the most important routine test. It is important to make sure that enough reliable measurements have been made to provide evidence good enough to allow an average blood pressure value to be calculated accurately, and thus to assess how big is the problem. Except in extreme emergencies at least three readings on separate days are necessary for this. For all but very severe cases, decisions on treatment can be made much better after two weeks of readings.

Once the doctor has made certain that the patient really have high blood pressure, he/she will investigate further. The investigation involves four main steps:

- An interview about medical history, current health and related activities
- A physical examination
- Routine test
- Other test

There are three principle reasons why one may need to have tests and investigations if he/she is found to have raised blood pressure levels:

- To check *cholesterol levels*. If both blood cholesterol level as well as blood pressure levels are high, the risk of developing heart disease and strokes is correspondingly greater, and thus treatment is required to bring both blood pressure and cholesterol levels back down to normal.

- To check for *serious underlying diseases*. Occasionally, high blood pressure may be caused by certain kidney diseases and some extremely rare diseases of the adrenal glands.

- To check for *heart and kidney damage*. This may occur after prolonged untreated high blood pressure. So tests are taken to measure kidney and heart affections.

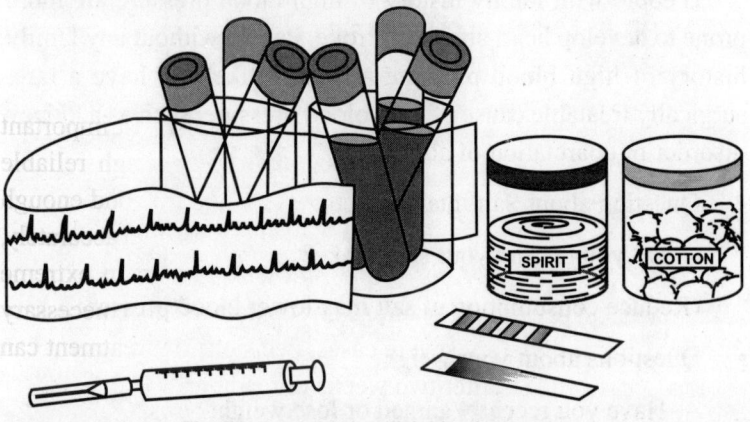

Fig. 21: Investigating high blood pressure

INTERVIEW (SAMPLE)

In an effort to determine future risk, doctors usually to ask some questions such as:

- Question about blood pressure measurements

   Doctors or nurses measuring blood pressure are all taught to look for reasons for unexpectedly high values. Was the blood pressure measurement likely to represent your normal blood pressure?

   —Did this measurement worry you?

   —Did you hurry for this appointment?

   —Do you have a full bladder?

   —Was there any other reason, any kind of discomfort or anxiety that might have pushed up blood pressure?

   (A rapid pulse is often due to anxiety or vigorous exercise within the previous 10–15 min.)

- Question about family

   —Were either of your parents or any of your brothers or sisters known to have high blood pressure?

   (People with family history of high blood pressure are more prone to develop heart attack or stroke. People without any family history of high blood pressure are more likely to have a rare, surgically treatable cause of high blood pressure, such as a kidney disorder or coarctation of aorta.)

- Question about Salt intake

   —Do you restrict your salt intake?

   (Reduce consumption of salt may lower blood pressure.)

- Questions about your weight

   —Have you recently gained or lose weight?

(If you are overweight for your height, it may cause high blood pressure. This is a readily treatable cause. Unplanned weight loss suggests thyroid or adrenal medulla hyperactivity.)

- Question about stress

    —Have you been under recent stress?

    (Recent stress may raise blood pressure and therefore blood pressure should be measured at less stressful time.)

- Questions about your drinking habits

    —How much alcohol do you drink per day?

    Drinking more than 4 units of alcohol a day for a man or 3 units a day for a woman is common cause of high blood pressure, particularly in people aged under 40.)

- Question about smoking

    —Do you smoke?

    (Regular smoking may increases the chance of heart and artery trouble and stroke.)

- Questions about exercise

    —Do you exercise?

    (Daily exercise is a healthy habit. It may reduce overall risk.)

- Questions about medications

    —Are you taking any medications?

    (Birth control pills, estrogen, diet pills and cold remedies may increase blood pressure. Again, this is an easily removable cause.)

- Questions about other diseases

    —Have you ever had a heart trouble or stroke?

    —Have you ever had any transient loss of vision, numbness or paralysis?

(History of heart attack or stroke is an effect of blood pressure on the body. Any transient loss of vision, numbness or paralysis is a warning of stroke. It shows effect of blood pressure on brain.)

PHYSICAL EXAMINATION

- **Height and weight**: If a person is overweight for his height it is considered as possible cause for high blood pressure. He is given advice to lose weight, which is likely to help reduce blood pressure.

- **Checking pulses:** In case of high blood pressure doctor checks the pulse not only at wrist but also at groin, feet and ankles.

The more severe the high blood pressure the smaller is amplitude of the pulse. Large amplitude i.e. the full, bounding pulse shows systolic high blood pressure (atherosclerosis) and not diastolic.

The pulse in feet and ankle provide information about the state of leg and coronary artery. Artery pulses below the inner side of the ankle and in the forefoot should be checked. The health of leg and coronary arteries in people above 40 yrs, should be assessed by taking these pulses and asking a few questions about legs. For example, if one regularly get pain in the calves or in front of chest after exercise such as prolonged walking, climbing stairs or hills, and these pains are worse in cold weather, or swelling in the feet, then this would suggest that the person might have some arterial problems.

A check on groin pulse and pulse at wrist showing no delay in pulse at groin, is enough to exclude a very rare condition called coarctation of the aorta.

- **Eye tests**: Damage to the eyes usually only occurs in people with very high pressure and so most people will need to have their eyes examined. People with very high blood pressure do need careful examination of retina, the doctor will probably use an instrument called an ophthalmoscope in a darkened room to look at the back of each eye (the retina). This is to look for swelling and bleeding around small retinal arteries which reveal imminent high risk of serious damage to the eyes, brain and kidney. In mild high blood pressure, these blood vessels show only very minor changes but in very severe high blood pressure there may be hemorrhage on the retina and areas of damage referred to as *cotton wool spots*. When found, this is a medical emergency requiring urgent attention.

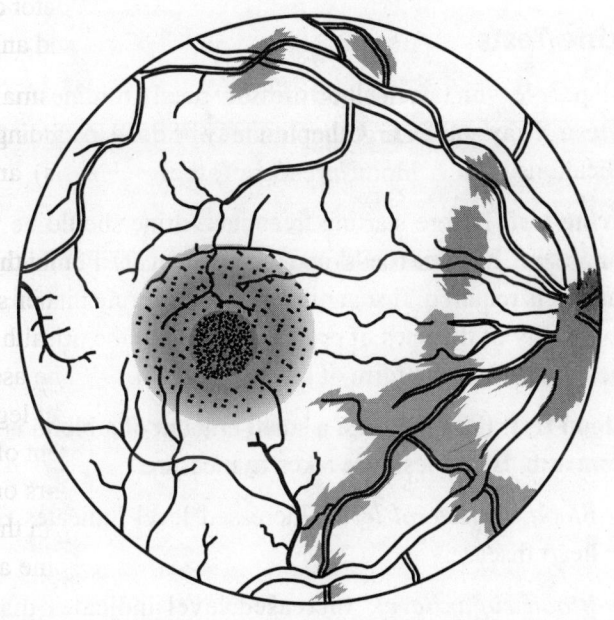

Fig. 22: Diagram of retina of a patient with hypertension

- **Heart and chest sounds**: Examination of heart and chest with a stethoscope may give some indication as to whether high blood pressure has affected heart. The type of heart damage called heart failure result in fluid retention that causes collection of fluid in the lungs which can be heard through a stethoscope. It can also cause enlargement of left side of the heart, which can be detected by the doctor.

Examination of heart and chest is only important for elderly people or those with pressure high enough to cause heart failure.

- **Listen to abdomen and neck**: While examining, listen to the sound of arteries of abdomen and neck. High pitch sounds indicate the narrowing of arteries to kidney, leg and brain respectively.

Routine Tests

All people with raised blood pressure need a routine urine test, blood test, X-ray and ECG. Other test may be done in case of some complications.

- **Urine test**: Before starting treatment, urine should be tested for protein, bacteria (cells) and glucose (sugar). For this a urine sample is required. If sugar is found in the urine this raises the possibility of diabetes, if protein is found in the urine it could mean there is some form of kidney problem.

- **Blood test**: For blood test a small amount of a blood is taken from arm. Blood tests are taken to measure:

    —*Blood cholesterol level:* Increased level indicates risk of heart disease.

    —*Blood sugar level:* Increased level indicates diabetes mellitus.

    —*Blood urea level:* It is raised in cases of kidney dysfunction.

    —*Blood creatinine level:* It is also raised in cases of kidney dysfunction.

—Level of sodium and potassium in blood: Levels are abnormal in people whose high blood pressure is due to retained sodium (high sodium and reduced blood potassium) because of the presence of a small benign tumor of the adrenal gland, this condition is called Conn's syndrome.

Sometime the doctor may ask for a number of other blood tests to be a carried out, that often gives clue to high alcohol intake—raised mean corpuscular volume, gamma-glutamyl transferase and triglyceride.

The result of these tests will provide a baseline measure for assessment of possible future organ damage and act as a check for possible cause.

- **X-ray**: At one time chest X-ray and special X-ray of the kidney (pyelography) were thought to be essential before starting treatment. But it is now known that these are not efficient ways of looking for secondary high blood pressure and so they are not necessary.

- **Electrocardiogram (ECG)**: Electrocardiogram (ECG) gives a recording of the electrical activity of the heart. An ECG has a dual purpose. First, it can provide an indirect index of the size of heart. When the blood pressure is very high, it enlarges in order to cope with increase load, this is called *left ventricular hypertrophy* (LVH) and is very important. When some one is found to have left ventricular hypertrophy, their need for treatment to lower their blood pressure becomes urgent because it indicates that the heart muscle is under significant strain and is trying to cope with the effort of pumping blood round the body at increased pressure. The second reason for doing an electrocardiogram is because it may show changes suggestive of narrowing or blockage of the coronary artery. This process is seen in people who experience chest pain (angina) on exertion. One single electrocardiogram trace is therefore a useful investigation for everyone before they start treatment for their high blood pressure.

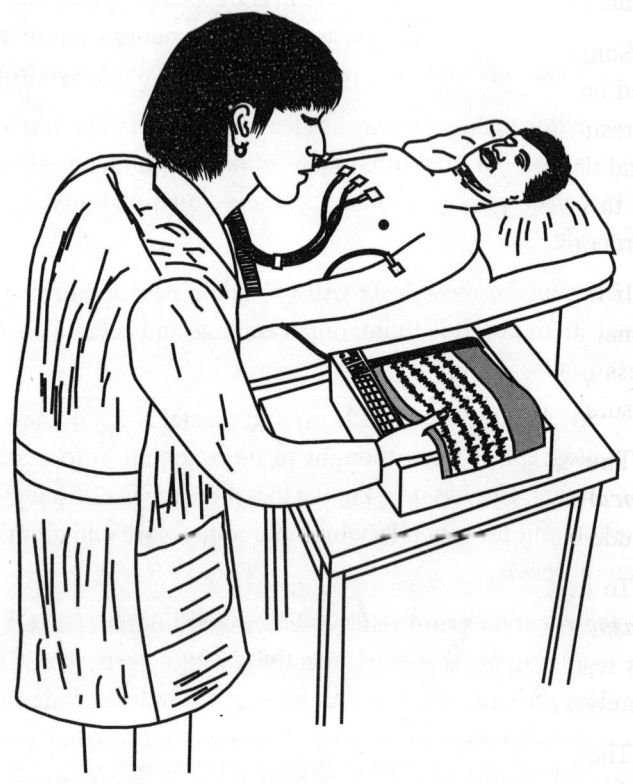

Fig. 23: Recording of ECG

- **Other tests**: Virtually everyone with high blood pressure will need the routine investigations mentioned above. More detailed investigations are required only if the blood pressure is severely high or if the doctor suspects some the underlying condition that is responsible for the blood pressure problem.

The vast majority of people with high blood pressure do not and should not need further investigations for their high blood pressure. Two or three percent of people with high blood pressure

Diagnosis and Investigations

are found to have underlying medical conditions that cause their blood pressure to rise. These are diseases of the kidney and of the adrenal gland.

Some underlying cause for the high blood pressure would be based on the presence of protein in the urine or abnormal blood test results, showing evidence of impairment of kidney function. In addition, if the level of potassium in the blood are found to be low, this raises the possibility that there may be an underlying disorder of the adrenal glands.

If there is a suspicion of Conn's syndrome (disorder of the adrenal gland), in which high blood pressure is the result of an excess of a hormone called aldosterone, the doctor may opt to measure this in patient's blood.

The doctor may also measure heart size by means of *echocardiogram*, which is a type of ultrasound heart scan, to exclude heart trouble.

To exclude any form of kidney disease, it is usual to do an *ultrasound scan* to investigate the size and shape of the kidney. This test is increasingly becoming a routine investigation for severely high blood pressure people.

There is a extremely rare condition called phaeochromocytoma that is caused by the intermittent secretion of large quantities of adrenaline and nor-adrenaline by a tumor of the adrenal gland. One may be asked to provide a **24-hour collection of** urine so that his body's 24-hour output of adrenaline and nor-adrenaline can be measured. Raised level could indicate *pheochromocytoma*.

In people with very high blood pressures or who already complain of symptoms suggesting minor stroke, i.e. transient giddiness, double vision, speech impairment, weakness of one side of the face or of one hand or of one leg and sudden loss of memory for recent events, brain damage can be assessed mainly by assessment of brain function. The most sensitive way to do this is to ask the person and their family the appropriate questions and **neurological tests** of eye movement, face or limb weakness, coordination, balance and various nerve reflexes. If these neurological test are done at all, they must be done well, which takes a long time.

■

Chapter 9

Management of High Blood Pressure

AIMS OF TREATMENT

It is known that high blood pressure is harmful. It shortens an individuals the life and increase the chance of having a heart attack, a stroke, permanent damage to the vision, damage to kidney or ballooning of the biggest artery. The high blood pressure is almost always 'silent' until above one of the mentioned complications occur. Almost everyone with high blood pressure has no symptoms until complications set in.

The only reason anyone needs treatment for high blood pressure is to prevent its likely consequences. All of the complications happen more often in people with uncontrolled high blood pressure—and the higher the pressure, the more likely they are to occur. The doctor recommends treatment for high blood pressure to reduce the risk of any of these unpleasant things in the future and to make one feel better today.

After treatment chances of developing any of these forms of organ damage should be much reduced.

High blood pressure is not the only cause of any of these kind of organ damage, so reducing the blood pressure cannot wholly prevent them. Smoking, high blood cholesterol levels and poorly controlled diabetes, which are often associated with overweight and insufficient regular exercise are another very important cause of all of them.

The treatment recommended will depend on how high the blood pressure is and what sought of lifestyle one has. The recommendation might be different, for example, for a younger person who is overweight, smokes, takes no exercise and has a blood pressure level that only needs to be brought down slightly than for someone much older who already leads a very healthy lifestyle and whose blood pressure needs to be brought down quiet a lot.

High blood pressure management consist mainly:

- Treatment without drugs
- Treatment with drugs:
    —With allopathic drugs
    —With homeopathic drugs
- Treatment with other alternative therapies

Chapter 10

Treatment without Drugs

If a person's blood pressure averages 160/105 mmHg or more, he will probably need some medication, whatever else he may do to bring his blood pressure down. Even so, person may need fewer drugs at a lower dosage if he modifies his lifestyle in some ways.

In this condition one should be able to bring down their blood pressure down by about 10 mmHg without needing drug treatment, just by modifying their lifestyle. It generally involves relatively straightforward changes of the diet and lifestyle. One may find it hard to make the necessary changes, it really is worth making a big effort. If the person is successful, his blood pressure may return to normal without the need for drug treatment. There are several ways in which one can help himself and really make a difference. There are five main areas where one may need to make changes in his lifestyle:

- Diet or healthy eating
- Weight control
- Exercise
- Smoking
- Alcohol intake (we will discuss it under the Diet)

DIET (OR HEALTHY EATING)

The goal of healthy eating is to discuss recommendations for diet that can help to control high blood pressure and reduce cardiovascular risk. Adjusting the foods that one eat will help keep blood pressure in check. The combination of high blood pressure and risk factors greatly increases the risk of developing cardiovascular disease.

Healthy eating is based on the following principles:
- A variety of food choices
- Emphasis on high fiber diet (cereals, breads and other grain products, vegetables and fruits)
- Reduce intake of fats and oils
- Reduce intake of salt
- High Potassium diet
- Limited alcohol
- Reduced caffeine

Healthy body weight can be achieved through a combination of healthy eating and regular exercise.

A Variety of Food Choices

A diet should be high in fiber, low in fat and salt. With these pointers in mind, emphasize fruits, vegetables and whole grains. Enhance the flavor of food with seasonings other than salt and avoid processed foods, which is high in sodium. One should also watch what he drink and keep cocktails to minimum.

On an average, vegetarians have lower blood pressure than meat eaters. Switching to a vegetarian diet lowers blood pressure in people whose BP is high enough to need treatment. Vegetarian diets have a high fiber content and high fiber foods are digested and absorbed slowly. They usually include plenty of pulses (peas, beans and lentils) which contain a particular type of fiber, called soluble fiber, which appears to lower blood cholesterol level. There is good evidence that the vitamins and minerals reduce blood pressure.

Potassium has one of the best record and this may be the main way in which a vegetarian diet works. Daily recommended is 3000–4000 mg per day which is found in abundance in fresh vegetables and fruits, especially bananas.

Calcium and **Magnesium** also helps to reduce blood pressure. One can obtain calcium naturally from nonfat or low-fat milk, yogurt and cheese. Many type of seeds, nuts, beans, peas and dark green leafy vegetables contain both calcium and magnesium.

Eat plenty of calcium rich food (minimum 1gm daily). Oils, fish, green vegetables, raw nuts and seeds, pulses and a little low-fat goats milk and cottage cheese are good source of calcium.

Calcium food values

Name	Total Calcium
1 cup of green vegetables	200–300 mg
103 nuts	80 mg
303 pulses	150 mg

Magnesium food value

Name	Total Magnesium
303 wholewheat bread	90 mg
303 brown rice	120 mg
303 soya beans	310 mg
303 nuts	80 mg
303 banana or dried fruit	80 mg

Spicy food may make face flush, but they have no effect at all on blood pressure.

Strict vegetarian diets can easily become deficient in protein, which is essential for building new cells. **Milk, cheese and other dairy products** are important sources of protein as well as variety for most vegetarian. Vegans, a group of vegetarians who eat no animal product at all, must rely on pulses, soya products and nuts for protein-rich foods. For reasons so far remain unexplained, people who drink a lot of milk tend to have lower blood cholesterol levels than people who drink little or none. Evidence for this is consistent and apparently reliable. However, milk does contain a lot of salt, and has to be restricted in low-sodium diet.

- **Egg yolk** is high in cholesterol. Prudent diets generally recommend not more than two eggs a week.
- **Fish** is a good source of fatty acids, which help relax arteries and thin the blood. Fish, particularly fish oil, have an important protective effect against coronary heart disease, and are therefore an important part of any prudent diet for people with high blood pressure. The effect is probably through omega-3 fish oils, which reduce blood levels of triglyceride.
- **Sugar** is important because it contains many calories and nothing but calories, so if one include a lot of sugar in his diet, he is more likely to put on weight. This is a good reason for avoiding foods high in sugar. However, there is no evidence that sugar of any kind has any specific harmful effect either on blood pressure or on the heart, or that eating sugar cause diabetes in any specific way other than contributing to energy imbalance: (calories in, calories out, don't eat more calories than you use, if energy in exceeds energy out, then surplus energy is stored as fat).
- Evidences show that **garlic** has no significant effect on high blood pressure, but it reduces blood cholesterol, and

therefore in turn reduces the risk associated with having high blood pressure.

The number of servings needed daily from different type of food varies depending on the age, body size, gender and activity. Healthy eating doesn't have to cost more. One can make changes in the diet gradually. This would in fact be better than doing it all at once, as it will give a chance to get accustomed to new eating habits and then one will be more likely to keep them up.

Emphasis on High Fiber Diet

Diet should be high in fiber and emphasis should be given to fruit, vegetables and whole grains in the diet. Blood pressure is lower in vegetarians than meat lovers. Vegetarian diet have a high fiber content and so it is digested and absorbed slowly, which means that one tends to feel full for long so its also useful in trying to lose weight.

Dietary fiber means everything in the food which cannot be digested, and which therefore passes through body until it is expelled in stool. Dietary fibre includes lots of important material which are required and affects the way in which food is absorbed, and the quantity in which it is taken to feel full.

Pulses (peas, beans and lentils) which contain a particular type of fiber-soluble fiber appear to lower blood cholesterol level. Pulses have the highest fiber content of any cooked vegetables.

Breakfast cereals, whole wheat bread, all fruit and vegetables have a high fiber content. Regularly adding sodium bicarbonate in cooking, to keep vegetable green rapidly destroys their fiber content and so does boiling them for a long time. Fresh fruits and raw salads are ideal.

Salads aren't compulsory. The important thing is to include plenty of fresh fruit and vegetables in diet, whether raw or cooked (don't overcook them). One can try different types of salads with different dressings on them (dressings that are low in fat but which still help to make even a simple vegetable/fruit taste better. For example, use olive oil dressing on salads, this will contribute monounsaturated fats to diet, and will thus be beneficial for heart).

Bread used to be the biggest single item in any ordinary person's life. All bread contain fairly high proportions of fiber, but whole wheat bread or granary loaves contain much more nutrients than ordinary bread and are therefore healthier. This is partly because one have to chew them more, which means that he will probably eat a bit less as they improve digestion of fat in the body.

One can increase the fiber content of food by eating more whole wheat bread, fruits and vegetables. This is one of the most effective steps one can take in any reduced fat, weight-reducing and cholesterol-lowering diet.

Reduce Intake of Salt

Sodium is one of the mineral which the body needs to keep functioning properly. While everybody needs sodium, most of the people eat far more than they need and could easily cut down without in any way damaging their health.

The main source of sodium in most foods is sodium chloride, which is the chemical name for ordinary cooking or table salt. Because salt is such a major source of sodium in diet, doctors often refer to reduce the amount of salt in the diet and thus automatically reduce the amount of sodium. Sodium is also found in other substances used in cooking and food processing, such as bicarbonate of soda (chemical name sodium bicarbonate) and monosodium glutamate (used in Chinese food and many sauces).

It has been thought that salt play an important role in the development of high blood pressure. Evidence to support this theory comes mostly from studying different populations of the world.

The studies show that primitive societies have a low sodium intake and a low incidence of high blood pressure. Western societies, however, have a high intake of sodium and increased rates of high blood pressure. In some tribes in Brazil and Papua—New Guinea, whose sodium intake is at the bare minimum essential for life, high blood pressure does not exist at all, nor does average blood pressure rise with age. On the other hand, in countries with very high sodium intake, such as rural Portugal or rural northern Japan, both high blood pressure and stroke are extremely common.

The studies did show that blood pressure goes up as salt intake increases. There are good biological reasons why sodium intake might affect blood pressure, mainly through its effect on the kidneys. The idea that salt overload is the cause of primary high blood pressure, with susceptibility to sodium overload genetically determined, seems quite likely. Evidence that substantial salt restriction is an effective or practical treatment for high blood pressure is much less convincing. What seemed to be more closely related to lower blood pressure was the dietary combination of *a lower salt* and *higher potassium intake*.

Only about one gram of the daily salt intake is added to food when it is on the table or during cooking. The rest major portion of salt comes mostly in tinned foods (such as vegetables), all ready prepared food (processed food) including burgers, pizzas, sausages, salted snacks, breakfast cereals, bread and in usually unsuspected foods such as milk and cheese.

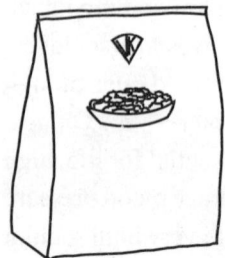 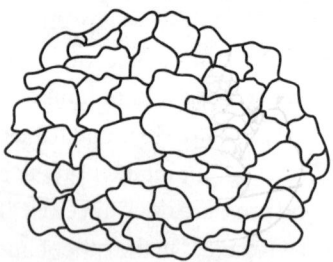

100gm breakfast cereals = 0.4 to 0.9gm

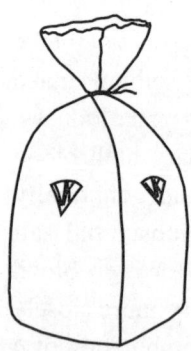 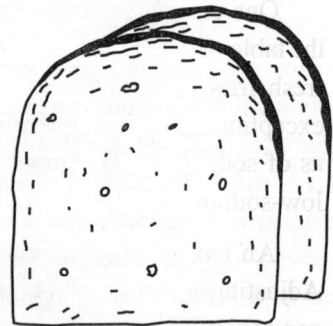

100gm wholemeal bread = 0.4 to 0.7gm

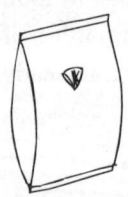 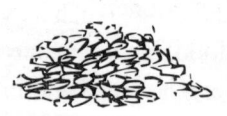 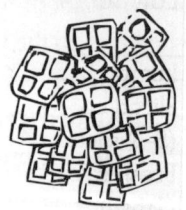

100gm salted snacks = 0.5 to 1.0gm

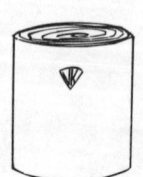 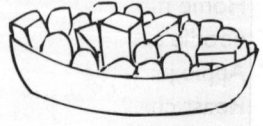

100gm tinned vegetables = 0.3 to 0.7gm

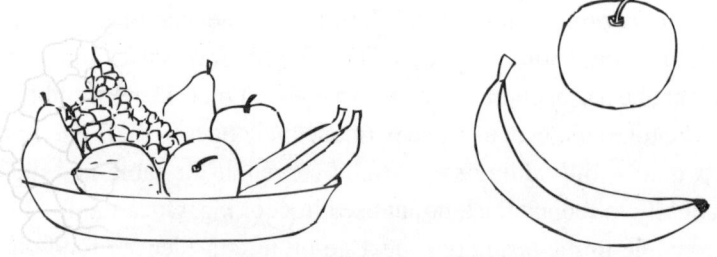

100gm fresh fruit = 0.1 to 0.2gm
Fig. 24: Diet: A variety of food choice for hypertensives

One can cut intake of salt by never adding salt to his food at the table or when cooking. Try to make more use of fresh meat and fresh fruit and vegetables, and only eat processed foods as the exception rather than the rule. Reducing the amount of fat as well as of sodium is very important because when a person follow a low-sodium diet, for the first few weeks all food tastes insipid.

An individuals taste preference for salt is an acquired habit. Adjusting to a low salt diet can be a little difficult at first but if one can consistently keep his salt intake down, then after a few months

Sodium Content of some commonly used food*			
Low Sodium	Sodium (mg)	High Sodium	Sodium (mg)
Lemon Juice (1tbsp)	0	Canned Salsa (1tbsp)	100
Sliced cucumber (5–7 slices)	4	Potato chips (10)	200
Fresh salsa unsalted (1tbsp)	5	Cheese spread	381
Plain popcorn (1c)	1	Canned corn (½c)	210
Frozen corn (½c)	3	Pizza slice	540
Home made chicken noodle soup (1c)	10	Plain hot dog with bun	866
Apple juice (8oz)	16	Large cheese burger	944
Roast chicken (2 slices)	32	Tomato juice	878
Roast beet sandwich	270	Soya sauce (1tbsp)	1029
		Pickles (1 large)	1428
*Value may vary with cooking methods			

he actually prefer his food with less salt. If one tend to go back to his old eating habits, he would find that his food tastes too salty and that he has become converted to low-salt diet. There should be a more tolerable way to make permanent changes in diet. The first step is to avoid adding salt to food served at the table and then gradually to reduce the amount used in cooking. Once the food is acceptable to the taste buds, next go on to consider the food one normally eats and workout what he should eat more, and what he should avoid.

Foods can be divided into three groups:

- Low sodium foods which one can eat as often as he likes
- 'Middling' sodium foods which one should eat sparingly
- High sodium foods which should be avoided altogether

Examples of foods from these groups are given here:

Low Sodium Foods

- All fresh fruits
- All fresh or home-cooked vegetables, but not cooked in sodium bicarbonate
- Fresh meat, fish and poultry
- Rice and pasta

'Middling' Sodium Foods

- Some milk and milk products—upto half a pint of skimmed or semi-skimmed milk a day; yogurt; cottage cheese; ice-cream
- Eggs not more than two a week
- Breakfast cereals—unsalted porridge, shredded wheat, puffed rice, wheat or oats
- Unsalted nuts
- Unsalted butter

High Sodium Foods

- Most snacks and fast foods – salted nuts, Bombay *bhelpuri*, *samosa*, *bhajias*, pizzas, pastries, burgers, peanut butter, fried chicken
- Tinned vegetables (including baked beans and tomatoes)
- Most milk products e.g. condensed milk, salted butter, all types of cheese except cottage cheese
- Smoked and tinned fish
- Preserved meats – this include ham, bacon and sausages
- Most breakfast cereals (all except those listed in 'middling' sodium foods)
- Curries
- Soup especially canned or packed soup (not home made soup)
- Dried fruits
- Chinese food
- Ordinary bread of any kind
- Ready-made sauces
- Biscuits and pastries
- Self-raising flour and baking powder
- Chocolate and toffees
- Saccharin

A dietician would be able to give more detailed information.

Decreasing your salt intake will allow one to get used to the taste of natural foods. Its surprising how good a fresh tomato taste without salt! If one want to add flavor to the food there are a number of herbs and spices which can be used. One can try seasoning your food with herbs and spices instead of vinegar. Mint and other herbs, mustard, pepper and other spices, and lemon juice can all be used on a low-sodium diet.

Cutting out the bicarbonate of soda while cooking would be an easy way to cut down sodium intake, as it has no effect on the taste of the vegetables. The 'soda' part of bicarbonate of soda is sodium. And using bicarbonate of soda when cooking vegetables destroys their vitamin C content, which is another good reason for leaving it out.

There is no advantage in using sea salt, rock salt and natural salt—they are still salt (that is, sodium chloride) and so are not salt substitutes. There are several **salt substitutes** now available at chemist shops. These contain less sodium chloride and more potassium chloride. Although, in an ideal world, no one should need to add crystals of any chemical substance to their food, if one really cannot tolerate food with a low-salt content he can use the salt substitutes instead, provided his kidney function has been shown to be normal.

High Potassium Diet

Populations who consume foods high in potassium have lower blood pressures. A diet rich in potassium is, by its very nature, also low in sodium. It is probably the combination of a low sodium and a high potassium diet that is most important in preventing the development of high blood pressure.

A potassium rich diet is especially important for people who are taking certain diuretics for their high blood pressure because these pills deplete the body's potassium.

Foods containing Potassium	
Excellent sources of Potassium (more than 500 mg/serving)	Good sources of Potassium (300–500 mg/serving)
Vegetables	**Vegetables**
1 cup (250 ml) pumpkins, spinach tomato or vegetable juice	1 cup (250 ml) broccoli, carrots, cauliflower, spinach, turnip, tomato, mushrooms
1 medium (100 gm) potato (baked potato skin)	1 medium (100 gm) sweet or potato (boiled)
Fruits	**Fruits**
1 medium (175 gm) banana 1 medium (340 gm) papaya 10 medium (100 gm) dates 1–4"×8" slice watermelon (925 gm) ½ medium (142 gm) avocado 10 halves (79 gm) dried avocado 5 halves (72 gm) dried peaches	1 medium (150 gm) orange ½ medium (241 gm) grape fruit 1 cup (250 ml) grape fruit, pineapple juice
	Milk
	1 cup (250 ml) whole milk, 2% skimmed buttermilk or goat milk
Seeds and Nuts	**Nuts and Lentils**
½c (125 ml) almonds and peanuts (shelled) or sunflower seeds	1 cup (250 ml) lentils 1 tbsp (15ml) peanuts butter ½ cup (125ml) cashew nuts
Beans and Peas	**Fish, meat, Liver**
1 cup (250ml) common white beans, soybeans, red kidney beans or split peas	90gm any cut of beef and pork (lean)

High potassium diets have been found to lower blood pressure in individuals being treated for high blood pressure. Increasing the amount of potassium in diet will not harm if one have normal kidney function. But if there is kidney disease, then the potassium intake should not be altered without consulting the doctor.

Although there is evidence that increasing the amount of potassium in the diet lowers the blood pressure, one should not take supplements in the form of potassium salts or tablets. Instead, one should increase the amount of potassium in diet by eating more fresh fruits and vegetables, and cutting the salt intake from processed foods at the same time.

Potassium intake can be increased by preparing foods in certain ways. Cooking in hot water has the effect of removing potassium. This can be prevented by cooking in a small amount of water and by leaving the skins on vegetables, cutting food into large pieces when boiling, and cooking until just tender. Save the cooking water to use in soups. Try steaming or baking the vegetables or use a microwave oven.

Reduced Intake of Fats and Oils

Fats are the most concentrated kind of energy available, so they contain more calories per gram than any other food. A diet high in fats or oils is therefore a diet high in energy. Most people consume more energy that they need and therefore gain weight, which is in turn another cause of raised BP.

Fats and oils are the main source of blood cholesterol. Although the cholesterol level does not directly affect the blood pressure, high blood cholesterol increases the chances of developing coronary heart disease and risk for stroke. Survey found that over half the people with high blood pressure also had an elevated blood cholesterol. The combination of these major risk factors increases the risk of heart diseases five-fold. Fats and oils differ only in their consistency. Fats are usually solid at room temperature, whereas oils are usually liquid. They all contain mixture of saturated and unsaturated fats.

Chemically fats and oils are made from long-chain molecules containing carbon, hydrogen and oxygen atoms. If there is no more space on the chain for any more oxygen atoms, then it is known as

saturated fat but; if there is space for more oxygen atoms, then it is known as **unsaturated fat**. Unsaturated fat are two types:

- **Monounsaturated** if there is room for only one more oxygen atom in the chain.
- **Polyunsaturated** if there is room for more than one oxygen atoms in the chain.

Saturated fats raise blood cholesterol, and thus the risk of heart disease much more than the unsaturated fats. Diet containing a higher proportion of unsaturated fats and oils are probably healthier. This is why one often hears that an oil or spread is 'high in unsaturates' or 'low in saturates'.

Saturated fats come mostly from animals example butter, coconut oil and palm oil are also high in saturates, and cheap cooking oil tend to include more saturated fats.

Unsaturated fats come mostly from vegetable oils or from animals fed on grass rather than grain. Vegetable oils high in polyunsaturated include corn, sunflower and soya oil. Olive oil is high in monounsaturated fats as are groundnut (peanut) oil and rape seed oil.

One should not only reduce total fat intake but also, where possible, switch from fats high in saturates to those high is unsaturates (and preferably high in monounsaturates rather than polyunsaturates).

If one is trying to loose weight, he may find a 'low-fat' spread (butter), but do remember that this will still contain a lot of calories and so should be used sparingly. In case of high blood cholesterol, one should change to a spread high in unsaturated fat-once again it should be remembered these still have the same total fat and calories content as butter, except that the saturated and unsaturated fats have been altered.

Recent research has shown that eating too much polyunsaturated fat can also be linked to the development of coronary heart disease. This mean that one will probably be better off switching to a spread high in monounsaturates.

Over 40% of the calories in an average diet comes from fats of various kind. To improve health, this level should be reduced to about 35% or less. People have greatly reduced their intake of milk, cream, butter but many other foods, for example snacks, fast food, etc. put the fat back.

The main aim is cutting down on fats, controlling blood cholesterol level should also be one of the goals. Here are some guidelines to help:

- Reduce total fat intake. Avoid high foods, frying or deep frying them or roasting them in fat.
- Limit the use of oil, butter, salad dressing, gravy and sauces
- Reduce intake of saturated fats from animal products such as meat, butter and cheese
- Choose lean cuts of meat and cut off any visible fat
- Remove skin from chicken and other poultry as most of their fat is in or just under the skin
- Skim any visible fat off the top of cooked dishes
- Replace high-fat food, e.g. Whole milk, cream, butter, high fat cheese, with their low-fat or reduced-fat equivalents e.g. skimmed or semi-skimmed milk, yogurt, low-fat butter, reduced-fat cheese
- Limit fat hidden in baked product and fast-food
- Cut down on snack foods which are often high in salt or sugar as well as in fats
- Cut down on biscuits, cakes and pastries, which all contain hidden fat—and lots of sugar
- Whenever possible, replace saturated fats or oil with monounsaturated or polyunsaturated fats or oils.

- Use moderate amounts of polyunsaturated fats such as corn, sunflower or soybean oils and monounsaturated fats like peanut (groundnut) oil or olive oil
- Limit high cholesterol foods including meats, organ meat, high fat dairy products, egg yolks, and butter
- Read the nutrition labels on food and choose those that have the lowest fat content
- Achieve a healthy body weight
- Increase fiber intake, especially foods high in soluble fiber such as dried peas, beans or lentils, fruit and vegetables, and whole grain products
- Exercise regularly
- Limit intake of sugar and alcohol

Limited Alcohol

There is good evidence that drinking only moderate amounts of alcohol maintains blood pressure and that one probably do not need to give up alcohol altogether. Recommended intake of alcohol is 21 units of alcohol per week for men and 14 units per week for women (one unit is equivalent to one small glass of wine or half a pint of beer or one single measure of spirit).

Drinking more than 4 units of alcohol a day for a men or 3 units of alcohol a day for a women is a common cause of high blood pressure, particularly in people aged under 40.

There is convincing evidence that drinking alcohol increases blood pressure. Drinking alcohol can lead to the development of high blood pressure in some individuals and may worsen the blood pressure in those who already have high blood pressure.

Acute heavy drinking (bingeing) can cause a rapid though brief rise in blood pressure, and this may bring on a stroke.

The good news is that having one or two drinks every day may be associated with lower levels of heart disease, probably through it effects on blood cholesterol and blood clotting factors. Heavier drinking increases the risk of high blood pressure and strokes, as well as having damaging effect on the liver, the nervous system and quality of life.

People whose diastolic pressure are over 100 mmHg due to drinking, can do without medication, once they reduce their drinking to not more than two units a day. High alcohol intake is a common cause of treatment failing to work, and if the blood pressure refuses to fall despite adequate treatment, one should think about what he is drinking.

WEIGHT CONTROL

Being overweight is a risk factor in the development of heart disease. Weight loss has also been found to reduce blood pressure in people who have high blood pressure. Being overweight is an important cause of high blood pressure particularly in young people under 40. It is important to note, however, that weight loss may not result in blood pressure lowering for some people, just as being overweight does not always mean that the blood pressure will be elevated.

For every kilogram of weight one looses, his blood pressure will fall by about 1 mmHg. So, if blood pressure is only slightly elevated, it may go down to normal if one manages to loose about 6 kg weight. This is not easy to do unless one is properly advised and strongly motivated. Weight loss will probably also reduce the risk of developing other health problems associated with being too fat, such as diabetes.

Everybody needs energy from food and drink to fuel their many body processes which must continue even when they are asleep.

All forms of physical activity such as walking, shopping, require additional energy. Energy is measured in calories. Ideally calorie intake from the food taken each day should balance the amount of energy used up by the body and when this happens one will neither gain nor loose weight. If the amount of food and drink one consume provides more energy than is used in daily activities, then the extra food will be converted into body fat and the person will put on weight. If one reduces daily intake of calories so that he is taking in less energy than his body needs, then the body uses its stored fat and he will loose weight.

To improve the general health, to reduce blood pressure and to lower the risk of coronary heart disease or stroke, to prevent or to improve control of diabetes, one require energy balance (calories in = calories out), which means taking more exercise as well as watching what he eats.

There is a better chance of reaching the target weight if one increases the amount of exercise he takes and cut down the alcohol he drinks. The combination of a sensible diet and regular exercise will build muscle and reduce fat stored. One should not be discouraged if he does not immediately seem to lose weight when following such a program—which you are replacing your fat with muscle, the change will not readily shown up on the weighing scales.

Recent research has shown that body shape is important. People who have their fat concentrated in the waist and abdomen, known as '**apple shape**' body, are more likely to develop high blood pressure and are at much higher risk of coronary disease than those overweight people whose excess fat is located mainly in theirs arms, thigh, and buttocks, known as '**pear shape**' body.

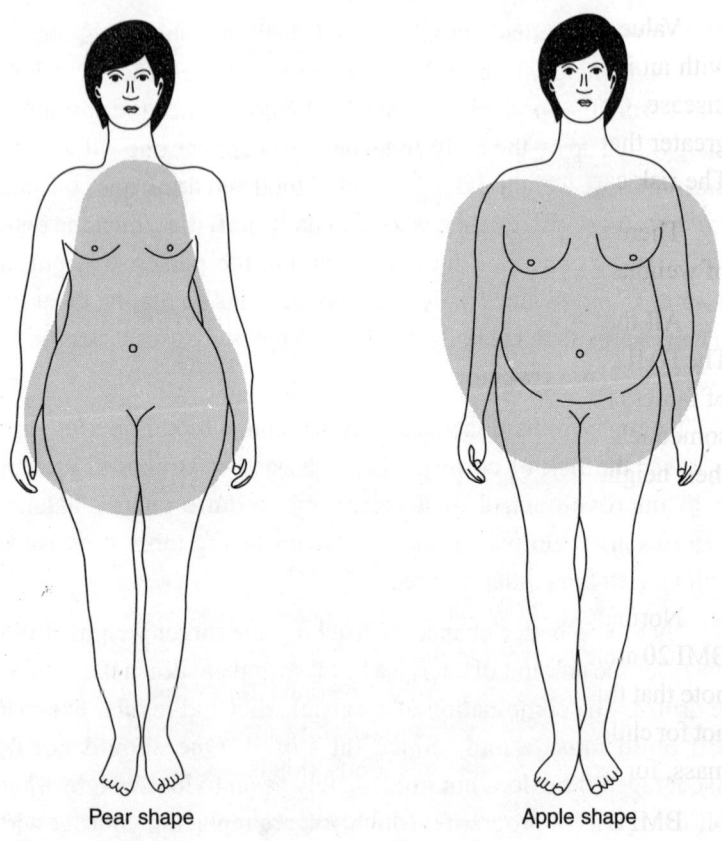

Fig. 25: Diagramatic representation of body shape due to fat concentration

The measure of distribution of body fat is referred to as a Waist to Hip Ratio (WHR). WHR can be calculated by dividing waist circumference by hip circumference, both at their widest point: a healthy result is less than 1.00. To measure waist circumference place the measuring tape at the point of waist narrowing, breathe out and measure to the nearest centimeter. For the hips, use the measurement of the largest bulge below the waist.

$$\text{Waist-to-Hip ratio (WHR)} = \frac{\text{Waist measurement}}{\text{Hip measurement}}$$

Value greater than 0.9 in males and 0.8 in females are associated with an increased risk of high blood pressure and cardiovascular disease. Coronary risk rise steeply in people whose belly girth is greater than their hip girth—the classical beer drinker's pot belly. The risk can be decreased by losing weight.

There are plenty of charts and tables which will show the range of weights that are considered average for the height.

All the adults aim for a body mass index (BMI) of 20 to 25. The BMI combines both height and weight to asses a person's level of fatness and includes weight from all body sources. To calculate someone's BMI, divide their weight in kilograms by the square of their height in meters.

$$BMI = \frac{\text{Weight in kilograms}}{(\text{Height in meters})^2}$$

Normal range of BMI is between 20 and 25. People below BMI 20 are underweight and above BMI 25 are overweight. Please note that this index applies only to adults 20 to 65 years of age but not for children, and does not make allowances for increased muscle mass, for example in athletes. Thus, this is only a guideline.

BMI is a good predictor for life expectancy. Very skinny people and very fat people both have lower than average life expectancy. The rise in death rates from obesity rises rapidly from a BMI of about 30, so this is a borderline between being overweight and serious obesity and BMI 40 as a borderline between serious obesity and giant obesity, which is very difficult to control.

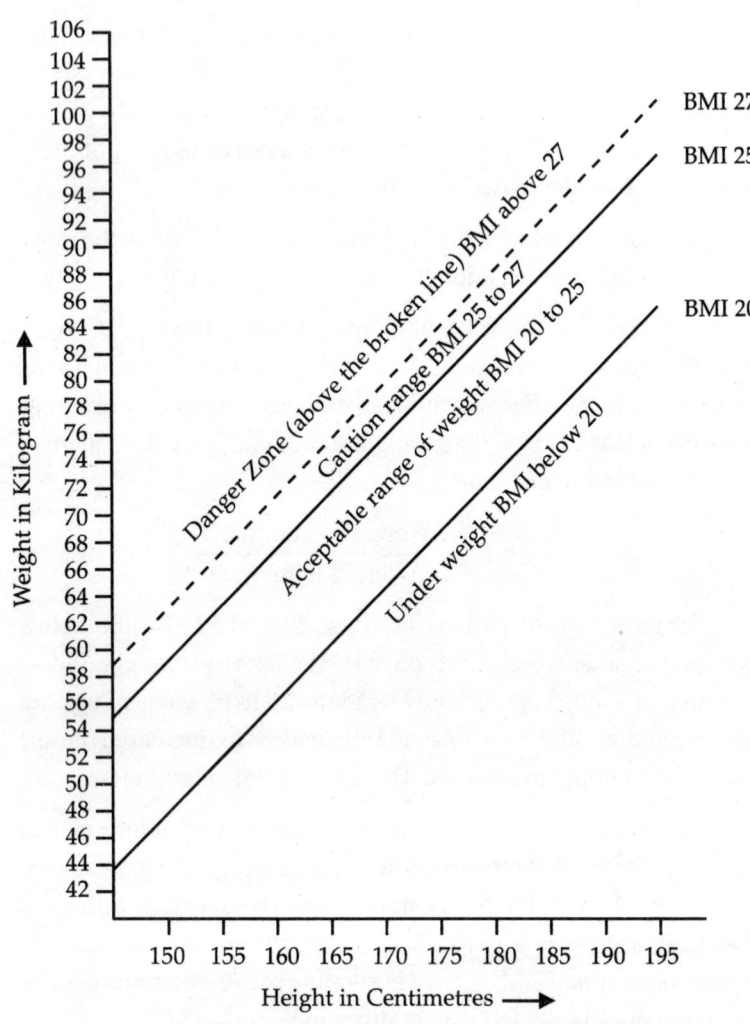

Fig. 26: Mesuring of the body mass index (BMI)

Sensible Weight Control

The most difficult part of any diet and exercise program is to keep up the morale and motivation. One should forget everything heard or read about quick weight loss schemes. There are no easy shortcuts. Because if one does that he will probably put all the weight back on again fairly quickly, as soon as he stops following his diet.

A slow weight loss is really the most efficient weight loss. There is plenty of evidence to show that people who lose weight quickly tend to put it all back on and more within just a few years.

Sensible weight control can only be achieved with consistent healthy eating habits and regular exercise. Maintaining these lifestyle changes will offer the greatest chance of success. The following are some of the golden rules:

1. **Set a realistic goal:** Losing weight slowly and steadily is the healthiest way to go about it. If one looses weight too fast he will not only loose his fat, but also the types of body tissue, such as muscles, that are essential. Start with a weight loss goal of a few pounds during a specific period of time, for example, lose ½ kilogram over a week or loose 2–4 kilogram over a month. The most important thing is simply to commit to a definite target, to weigh oneself once a month or once a week on reliable scales and to be honest about the results.

2. **Take regular exercise:** Participate in some form of regular exercise for at least 30 minutes a day, at least three to four times a week. This doesn't have to be strenuous exercise, but one does need to move his large muscles, especially the legs. A regular walking program have helped many people achieve and maintain weight loss. Any kind of exercise can help one lose weight. For example take the stairs instead of the elevator.

   Remember that losing weight on a calorie—reduced diet but without exercise program will have less effect on the blood pressure than the same weight loss achieved with an exercise program.

3. **Eat less fat:** Fats are the most concentrated kind of energy available, so they contain more calories per gram than any food. A diet high in fats or oils is therefore a diet high in calories.

People become overweight because they are eating too much fat and not using it up through exercise. Switch to skimmed or partially skimmed milk and decrease intake of butter, salad dressing and mayonnaise. Trim the fat from meats and the skin from poultry. You will find more information about this in the section of **reduce fats and oils** earlier in this chapter.

4. **Eat regular meals, stop munching:** Eat regular meals. Skipping meals can lead to binge eating and make is harder to maintain any weight lose. Body prefers to have a regular supply of food, so do not be tempted to go over the top and miss meals altogether. It one does, he will either eat too much at your next meal to make up for it, or may even develop an obsessive relationship with food which will be certainly bad for health and could even lead to eating disorders such as anorexia or bulimia.

   Munching between meals can add a lot of surplus calories to an individual's diet without noticing, especially as many snack foods are high in fats or sugar. So one of the best things to do is to stop munching. If one really do need a snack, then a piece of fruit is probably the best choice.

5. **Eat more fiber content:** Increase the fiber content in diet. Fiber helps to keep one from feeling hungry between meals. Whole grain products such as bread, fruits, vegetable, and legumes are high fiber sources. Reducing the amount of fats and sweet foods from the diet is easier if they are replaced by those foods that contain less energy. They are generally more bulky and need more chewing and are also digested more slowly, helping one to feel full for longer time. They also provide the vitamins and minerals that are essential in a healthy diet.

6. **Eat less sugar:** Reducing the amount of sugar one eat helps in reducing the calorie intake. Sugar has no nutritional value as it

contains nothing but calories, whether one eats it on its own or in sweets, honey and soft drink, biscuits, cakes, or hidden in processed foods.

7. **Eat in moderation:** Diet involving severe calorie restriction rarely works for the long term. As hunger is a strong physiological desire, the body responds to calorie restriction as if starvation were at hand. The eventual result is binge eating and the potential for greater fat storage. Choose healthy foods and eating just until satisfied will enable one to lose weight more successfully. Intake of sugar, sweets and alcohol should be moderate.

8. **Weight measurements:** Measure the weight honestly and regularly on accurate scale. A good set of weighing scales is important one as looses weight slowly at a rate of ½ kilogram a week, and these amounts need to be measured accurately. Ordinary weighing scales vary from hour to hour and day to day, depending on temperature and humidity. One should stick to more or less the same clothes each time one weigh and should not bother to weigh himself more than once a week.

If one follows these rules, he will be eating a healthy diet, and you will lose weight without consuming expensive 'diet' food or having to count each individual calories.

EXERCISE

People who lead inactive lifestyles are much more likely to have high blood pressure. Participating in regular exercise not only helps us to stay in shape and maintain a normal body weight but can also actively lower blood pressure. Research has proved that there is a clear association between taking more exercise and a fall in blood pressure. The long-term effect of regular exercise is to reduce diastolic blood pressure by 10 mmHg. Regular exercise also reduces a wide range of important risk factors for coronary heart disease and stroke. It not only reduces harmful LDL and VDL blood cholesterol levels but also raises HDL blood cholesterol. It also reduces levels of the blood clotting factor fibrinogen. Regular exercise often helps people to stop smoking due to its feel-good effect.

If one has high blood pressure then it would be wise to consult the doctor before deciding on the exercise programme. For example, for an overweight middle-aged man with severe high blood pressure who have never taken any exercise it would be unwise to take up vigorous exercise that leaves him feeling exhausted. The immediate effect of vigorous exercise is to raise blood pressure. The rise is part of body's process for preparing and sustaining the individual through exercise, because while exercising one you need an increase in blood flow to the large muscles in the body. But the rise only last for a short period. It is much better to opt for a graded programme of gradually increasing exercise. First, one must be willing to become more physically active in everyday life.

Moderate exercise works—for example getting off the bus one stop earlier and walking the remaining distance to the destination or simply walking on short journeys rather than driving will be good for blood pressure. Use of stair case instead of the elevators or getting off the elevator one floor earlier will also be effective. Any form of sport is fine provided one does not exhaust himself.

One can probably think of many other methods to increase routine exercise with the tight schedules of life and you may have to make some minor concessions to change his exercise habits. On the other hand, one may find that walking for 30 minutes in the evening before dinner becomes an enjoyable part of the day.

Just how much exercise is needed to bring down blood pressure and improve general health will depend on many factors:

- Age
- How fit the person is?

- How much exercise a person can take?
- Whether he/she has any problems in addition to high blood pressure, and many more

People with high blood pressure need to choose a form of exercise which is dynamic. This gives you plenty to choose from:

- Walking
- Running
- Swimming
- Cycling
- Dancing

The first rule of all successful exercise programs is for people to do what they want, what interests them.

Walking: Walking is simple and cheap, all one needs is some comfortable shoes. It is easy to introduce into daily routine. One can get as much benefit walking briskly in the local parks or around local towns.

Swimming: Swimming is good form of exercise for all age groups. It is an ideal form of exercise especially for older people or people with arthritis because body is weightless in water, the water supports weights, and movements may become almost painless when one is immersed in water.

Running or Jogging: It seems to appeal most people who like their own company. One will need proper running shoes otherwise he may damage his feet, ankles or knees.

Cycling: Cycling is excellent exercise for everyone except people with back problems.

Dancing: Dancing appeals to people who enjoy exercising to music. It can be any type of dancing, be it rock 'n' roll, jazz, ballroom, country dancing whatever.

Whatever exercise one may choose, start slowly and train up gradually. As a rule of thumb **most people will need to aim for 20–30 minutes of moderate exercise about three times a week**. If a significant antihypertensive effect of exercise become evident, the doctor may want to postpone or modify drug treatment.

What to avoid: If one has established high blood pressure he should avoid extremely vigorous sports such as squash and also static exercises such as weight lifting and push-ups, all of which may briefly raise his blood pressure to dangerous level.

The goal should be to change lifestyle, from sedentary to more active. It is not possible to achieve this overnight! Be patient and persistent.

SMOKING

Smoking does not cause high blood pressure, but it greatly increases the risks of other diseases that go with having high blood pressure. People who already have high blood pressure are three times more susceptible to a heart attack due to smoking up to about 50 years of age, and chances are doubled after that age. Smoking is a very powerful risk factor not only for coronary heart disease and stroke, but also for cancer of the mouth, throat, nose, lung, larynx, bladder and pancreas, for asthma, and other obstructive lung disease and for obstructed leg arteries. Heart attack in people under 45 years of age, happens almost entirely in smokers.

Stopping smoking in people with high blood pressure reduces the risk of coronary heart attack more than reducing blood pressure. Stopping smoking also reduces the risk of many other serious problems.

The aim of treating high blood pressure is not to reduce the pressure for its own sake, but to reduce the risks of having high blood pressure. People will achieve health gains if they can stop smoking and reduce blood pressure.

Some allopathy drugs such as Beta blocker drugs, which are often used to reduce blood pressure, seem to be less effective in people who continue to smoke. They still reduce blood pressure, but fail to reduce the risks of heart disease.

It is not easy to quit smoking. There are many helpful aids and programs to help quit smoking these days, including nicotine replacement therapy. If one find it difficult to stop smoking on its own, doctor can help him or refer him to special clinics or programs.

People start smoking for many reasons and continue smoking as a habit. It's worth discussing reasons with someone who is experienced in helping people to stop smoking. Temporary substitution of nicotine by another less dangerous route can be a big help in stopping smoking. This can be done by many techniques like chewing tobacco or using nicotine chewing gum. Although all these techniques are often effective one need to remember that his ultimate aim is to stop taking nicotine altogether. If an individual goes on taking more or less the same amount of nicotine by these other routes, he will not reduce his risk of coronary heart disease.

Chapter 11

Treatment with Drugs

While essential high blood pressure can be treated effectively, the secondary high blood pressure can often be cured by addressing the underlying cause. One can do a number of things to control his high blood pressure—but should consult a physician before he gets started.

Most doctors prefer to suggest lifestyle changes before prescribing drugs. A comprehensive lifestyle program will include dietary changes that promote nutrition and lower salt intake, regular aerobic exercise, weight loss and a ban on smoking.

Some high blood pressure cases require drug therapy, either because of their severity or because they have failed to respond to self-help measures. A person need drug therapy if:

- There is already evidence of organ damage for example, angina, or stroke or arterial leg pain
- He also has diabetes
- His average BP is around 160/110 mmHg or more

Drug therapy includes:

- Allopathy drugs

- Homeopathy drugs
- Other alternative therapies

TREATMENT WITH ALLOPATHY DRUGS

Before 1950, there was no practical way to lower blood pressure with or without medication. In the last 55 years, hypertensive drugs became available and lowered blood pressure and did save lives. Many of those early drugs, which are no longer used, were however associated with severe side-effects. Between 1950 and 1970, most of the attention was directed towards patients with more severe high blood pressure because drugs often caused troublesome side-effects. During the 1970s, drugs with fewer and less dramatic side-effects became available and these could therefore be given to people with milder high blood pressure who were at a lower cardiovascular risk.

The development of antihypertensive drugs with minimal side-effects and their immense benefits in terms of prevention of heart attacks and strokes had been one of the biggest advances in medical care. Antihypertensive drugs have also been shown to be effective in reducing or preventing kidney damage in people with diabetes, and more recently some drugs prevent damage to the retinas of people with diabetes.

GOAL OF TREATMENT

The only reason anyone needs treatment for high blood pressure is to prevent its likely consequences. The good news is that careful treatment works. After treatment, chances of developing any form of organ damage should be much reduced. It has left no more room for doubt that anybody with high blood pressure should be left without treatment for more than a few weeks.

It is known that lowering blood pressure to less than 150/90 mmHg will reduce complications. Very generally speaking, treatment usually aims at a target below 140/90 mmHg. If it can be maintained below 140/85 mmHg, so much the better. However, there is less certain it about the best blood pressure to aim for. In most cases, the goal is to lower blood pressure to less than 140/90 mmHg. The goal differs in the elderly with systolic pressure, in their case, the threshold for beginning therapy should be a little higher than 160/90 mmHg. It is now, however, true to say that the complications of high blood pressure would be avoidable if blood pressure can be controlled.

If the average blood pressure over a whole three month period is 150/90 mmHg or higher, then one probably need BP—lowering drugs.

The treatment recommended for high blood pressure will depend on how high blood pressure is and what sought of lifestyle person have. The recommendations might be different, for example, for a younger person who is overweight, smokes, takes no exercise and has a blood pressure level that only needs to be brought down slightly than for someone much older who already leads a very healthy lifestyle and whose blood pressure needs to be brought down quiet a lot.

CONTROLLING BLOOD PRESSURE BY DRUGS

All the blood pressure lowering drugs manipulate, in various ways the body mechanisms which normally control distribution of blood flow between different organs. Blood pressure can be lowered by reducing the total volume of blood in the body, by relaxing the spiral muscles around small arteries and thus widening their diameter, or by reducing heart output. All the drugs now in use operate through one or more of these final pathways, but they vary greatly in the way they reach them. Some act first on the brain, some on different functions of the kidney, some directly on the heart or small arteries.

All drugs that lower blood pressure are roughly equally effective. They drop the systolic pressure by about 10–15 mmHg and the diastolic pressure by 6–8 mmHg. If one is on drug therapy, he should also remember that the effect of some drugs is greater if he reduces his salt intake.

Blood pressure lowering drugs have also been shown to be effective in reducing or preventing kidney damage in people with diabetes, and more recently some drugs have been shown to prevent damage to the retinas of people with diabetes. It is now, however, true to say that the complications of high blood pressure can be avoided if blood pressure is controlled.

Individual responses to blood pressure lowering drugs are often surprising, some people with very high blood pressure gets a large fall with only a small dose of one drug, while others still have poor control despite full dosage of two or even three. Blood pressure lowering drugs are from different groups. A person can start two different blood pressure lowering drugs at the same time. But it seems more sensible always to start drugs one at a time. If two different medicine are started at the same time and if there is some unpleasant side effect, it won't be known which drug is causing it.

If a person's blood pressure really has always been well below target pressure for several years, he should discuss with his doctor whether it is worth while considering doing without drugs for a trial period. It is very unlikely that anybody will ever be able to stop their drug completely, although they may well manage with simpler medication and/or a lower dose. A few people, rightly treated for definitely raised blood pressure when in their 30s, seem to be able to stop taking medication after many years of good control without returning to their original high pressure, but this seems unusual.

Any attempts to do without drugs should be undertaken cautiously, with close supervision. If doctor decides to go ahead, taper off the tablets (don't suddenly stop taking tablets), then the patient should have weekly blood pressure checks for the first month, then monthly checks.

Side-effects of Drugs

There are very few drugs which have no side-effects at all and blood pressure lowering drugs are no exception. The different groups of drugs have different possible side-effects. There are two side-effects which are common to several groups of blood pressure lowering drugs. The first is **impotence**—all blood pressure lowering drugs can occasionally cause partial or complete failure of erection in men. The effect is reversible. The second is **fainting**—a few blood pressure lowering drugs can cause either feeling of faintness, or an actual faint with momentary unconsciousness. Faints occur because of sudden drop in blood pressure, so that blood supply to the brain falls below the level necessary to maintain consciousness. If one sit down with his head between his legs for a couple of minutes, the faint can be avoided. It is quite likely that some of these effects are inseparable from reduction in blood pressure.

Important Tips on Drug Treatment

Until recently high blood pressure was generally considered only to be a disease of people in older age groups. And it was uncommon for younger people to have their blood pressure checked. This practice is now changing. Now it is a fairly common disease in young adults. The **young adults** should not ignore their high blood pressure or take it lightly. Many young adult had developed some of unpleasant consequences of high blood pressure by the time they reached 40, because they are not taking any medication for their high blood pressure. Many of these unpleasant consequences could have been avoided it they had started on blood pressure lowering drugs at a younger age.

The ways of treating high blood pressure in young adults without medication must be considered and usually tried seriously. For overweight young adults, there is now good evidence that effective weight reduction combined with a regular exercise programme reduce blood pressure as much as usual blood pressure lowering medication. But both weight control and exercise have to be kept up indefinitely. If blood pressure does not fall after about six months of serious effort in young adults, then blood pressure lowering drugs needs to be considered.

People of **old age** (65 year and above) tolerate all drugs less well than younger people because their kidney and liver eliminate drugs less efficiently and their bodies are generally less able to tolerate big changes, including changes in blood pressure. On the other hand, elderly people generally respond to blood pressure lowering drugs just as well as younger people, perhaps rather more so. They often show a good fall in blood pressure with smaller dose of blood pressure-lowering drugs than are required by middle-aged people.

Blood pressure lowering medications should never be stopped abruptly, because this can cause a steep 'rebound' rise in blood pressure, to even higher levels than before treatment started, with a serious risk of bringing on a stroke or heart attack.

Some blood pressure lowering drugs are more effective if person reduces the amount of sodium in his diet substantially. The same dose will then have a greater effect on blood pressure, or one will be able to get the same effect from a lower dose.

If you are convinced your medication is making you ill, see your doctor as soon as possible and ask it you can stop taking it and change to a different drug.

All slow release (SR) drugs are designed to be taken either with a meal or soon after. Otherwise, timing in relation to meals is unimportant, except that a fixed routine is easier to remember.

Different Drugs for High Blood Pressure

There is now a wide choice of blood pressure-lowering drugs. Manufacturers introduce new drugs and withdraw older ones all the time so the drugs come and go from the market very rapidly.

All the drugs have two names:

- The **generic name** or scientific name is the name given to each drug when it is first developed.

- The **brand name** or trade name is the name given to a drug when it is manufactured by a drug company.

Different Groups

Blood pressure lowering drugs can be divided into 10 groups according to the mode of action.

There are usually so many different drugs and brands in each groups with few significant differences between them, that it may be safely assumed that whatever is said about the group applies equally to all drugs included within it.

The groups are presented in the order of general preferences, starting and ending with those least likely.

Groups in General Order of Preference

First line drugs

Group 1 Diuretics

1A Thiazide and thiazide-like diuretic

1B Potassium sparing diuretics

1C Diuretics with potassium supplement

1D Loop diuretics

Second line drugs

Group 2 Beta-blockers

Third line drugs

Group 3 Angiotensin converting Enzyme (ACE) inhibitors

Group 4 Angiotensin inhibitors

Group 5 Vasodilators

Group 6 Alpha-blockers

Group 7 Calcium-channel blockers

Forth line drugs

Group of Drugs acting mainly on the brain stem.

Last line drugs

Group 9 Adrenergic neuron blockers

Group 10 Ganglion blockers

Many patient can be satisfactorily treated with a single blood pressure-lowering drug, the choice of which will be determined by safety, convenience and freedom from side effects. Another large group will require a combination of two or three blood pressure-lowering drug to give good control with minimum of side effects.

Group 1: Diuretics

They were first introduced in 1950's. Diuretics are available in four subgroups. Of these, only those in thiazide diuretics are generally useful for treating high blood pressure and they are the drugs most commonly used today. Use of other drugs should be avoided.

The main purpose of diuretics is to increase urine output. For this reason they are often known as 'water tablets'. The main action by which diuretics reduces blood pressure is probably by increasing output of sodium through the kidneys, although they also widen small arteries and reduce blood volume. These drugs are very effective blood pressure lowering drugs. Their action is more effective if person also reduces his salt intake. These drugs work

Treatment with Drugs

by widening blood vessels and helping the kidney to get rid of salt and water in urine.

- **1A Thiazide diuretics**: Thiazides have their blood pressure lowering effect in very low doses: if it is consumed more than this, it greatly increase the risk of side effect, without any advantage in reducing blood pressure.

Thiazide diuretics reduces the excretion of calcium through the kidney therefore it reduces the tendency of stone formation in the kidney. In addition, it reduces tendency to develop osteoporosis (bones become brittle) after menopause in women.

Common Thiazide Diuretics:

- Bendrofluazide
- Chlorthfidone
- Chlorothiazide
- Hydrochlorothiazide
- Metruside
- Metolazone
- Cyclopenthiazide
- Polythiazide
- Indapamide
- Xipamide
- 1 B Potassium sparing diuretics
- 1C diuretics with Potassium supplements

Low blood potassium was thought to be a common side-effect of diuretics given for high blood pressure. This concern led to the development and promotion of the following two groups of drugs. **The potassium sparing diuretics**; were intended to prevent excessive potassium loss. **The potassium supplement diuretics**; were intended to replace any potassium that had been lost.

No drug of these groups should be used routinely for high blood pressure treatment because they can lead to increased level of potassium in body, known as hyperkalaemia.

- **1D Loop diuretics**: Loop diuretics push sodium and water out of the kidneys more powerfully than thiazide diuretics, but they are much less effective in lowering blood pressure.

Side-effect of Thiazide Diuretics:

- Thiazide can cause impotency when prescribed in large doses
- They should not be used in pregnancy because they cross the placenta and therefore reach the unborn baby
- The two common side effect at the low dose are gout and diabetes. Diuretics sometimes cause an increase in uric acid and can start an attack of gout in those who have a tendency to it.
- They are known to cause dangerous fall in blood potassium levels

At least half of all people with high blood pressure were treated by combining two drugs from different groups, usually thiazide diuretic plus something else

The thiazide diuretics at low doses are almost always the first choice in old age group

Group 2: Beta-blockers

Beta-blockers work mainly by blocking transmission of nerve messages from the brainstem to the spiral muscle sheath around the small arteries, via blocking the action of noradrenaline that together with another chemical called adrenaline, prepares the body for emergency situations (flight or fight response). These powerful hormone open some blood vessels and narrow others, controlling blood flow to vital organs such as heart. Noradrenaline and adrenaline also speed up the action of heart, make it pump more forcibly and raises the blood pressure. Beta-blockers stop all this through blocking the action of noradrenaline and adrenaline and so slow down the heart, lessen the force of its contractions and lower blood pressure. However, they also narrow the airways in the lungs, so it cannot be taken in asthmatic individuals. As they lessen the force of the heart's contractions, they may not be suitable if heart is not pumping well anyway.

After the thiazide diuretics, these have been the most commonly prescribed group of blood pressure-lowering drugs since past 15 years. Although, the ACE-inhibitors are now catching them up.

Beta-blockers has a calming effect on nervous people. Beta-blockers have been used successfully to control nervousness in public speakers, in people who drive and other similar stressful events. Beta-blockers are also very effective in preventing attacks of angina.

Common Beta-blockers Drugs:

- Nadolol
- Pindolol
- Celiprolol hydrochloride
- Metoprolol tartrat
- Sotalol hydrochloride
- Oxprenolol hydrochloride
- Labetalol hydrochloride
- Esmolol hydrochloride
- Timolol maleate

Side-effects of Beta-blockers Drugs:

- Serious side-effect is that these narrow lung airways in people. Because of this effect, even a single dose of a beta-blocker can be dangerous for people with asthma.

- On a long-term basis, they may subtly reduce energy level as they make heart pump less forcibly and more slowly. That way some people feel tiredness and a generally reduced level of energy and athletes or people doing heavy manual work may notice that they become fatigued more quickly.
- They may cause cold hands and feet because they reduce the output from the heart
- Few like propranolol, which reach the brains can cause vivid dreams and sleep disturbance
- They may cause problem of temporary impotence in some men but it is reversible
- If used earlier in pregnancy, they may slow down the baby's growth and so should be avoided, but they can be used after 24th week of pregnancy.
- Much rarer but serious side-effect is further reduction in heart output in people who have heart failure or who are on the verge of heart failure.

Group 3: Angiotensin Converting Enzyme (ACE) Inhibitors

ACE inhibitors were first introduced in 1981. These are the most recently introduced major group of blood pressure-lowering drugs currently in common use. They are already the first choice of many doctors for routine treatment indicates. These drugs may be particularly useful for treating the majority of people who need to start drug treatment under age 40. Not only do these drugs lower blood pressure, but they also protect the kidneys of people with diabetes and high blood pressure. Recently, they have been shown to delay the onset of retinal damage, which can impair the vision of people with diabetes.

Angiotensin II constricts blood vessels. ACE inhibitors work by preventing the activation of the hormone angiotensin II from its two precursors, rennin and angiotensin I. Because angiotensin II constricts blood vessels, resulting in lowering of blood pressure. They increase salt excretion by the kidneys when it is too much in the body and conserves it when there is not enough. This means that the normal mechanisms for correcting sudden fluid and salt loss cannot operate in people taking these drugs, which can cause serious problems if an attack of severe diarrhoea and/or vomiting leads to dehydration. One will need to drink large quantities of extra water with one teaspoon of salt and one teaspoon of sugar added to each litre of water.

The ACE inhibitors are started in people who are already taking thiazide diuretics. These people need to be monitored closely because the first dose can cause a sudden fall in blood pressure and there is a risk that collapse may occur in cases of kidney failure. People already taking thiazide diuretics are advised to stop diuretic and leave at least 4–5 days before starting ACE inhibitors. ACE inhibitors are very effective in the treatment of congestive heart failure. They seem to be effective and trouble free in treatment of high blood pressure at old age.

Common ACE-inhibitor Drugs:

- Captopril
- Fosinopril
- Ramipril
- Quinapril
- Lisinopril
- Cilazapril
- Perindopril
- Trandolapril
- Enalapril maleate
- Moexipril hydrochloride

Side-effects of ACE-inhibitors:

- The commonest side-effect of the ACE-inhibitors is a dry chronic irritating cough, which affects 25% of the people who take them, 10 percent in men and 20 percent in women
- Captopril causes a bitter or salty taste in the mouth in about 20% of the people who take it. The taste disappears in about 14 days after stopping the drugs.
- An acute allergic response to this type of drug—tongue and lips swell and their upper airways become constricted. This happens rarely
- ACE-inhibitors should be avoided in pregnancy because they affect the baby's blood pressure may impair the development of the baby's skull and may reduce the volume of amniotic fluid

Group 4: Angiotensin II Receptor Antagonists

Angiotensin II Receptor antagonists first introduced in 1994. These descendants of ACE-inhibitors are often called ACE II agent with the first generation of (ACE-inhibitors) called ACE I. These work in a similar manner as ACE inhibitors, by blocking the angiotensin converting enzyme inhibitors. The action of angiotensin II is that if causes arterioles to constrict because the mechanism is not direct. Angiotensin II stockers, may cause fewer side effects.

They lower blood pressure effectively and have been proved remarkably safe. They do not cause troublesome side-effects such as a cough. They are useful for people who get a persistent dry cough with first-generation ACE-inhibitors.

Angiotensin receptor antagonists share many actions with the ACE-inhibitors and some of the actions of the Beta-blockers. For this reason, they might be expected to work less efficiently for older people and those of Aero-Caribbean origin.

Common Angiotensin II Receptor Antagonist Drugs:
- Losartan potassium
- Valsartan
- Candersatan cilexetil
- Albertan

Group 5: Vasodilators

These drugs reduce blood pressure by relaxing the arteries and increasing their diameter (dilate the lumen). If this dilation was the only effect, these drugs would be well suited for the treatment of high blood pressure. But they tend to increase heart rate and heart output unless they are combined with beta-blockers. Minoxidil is the last-restort drug for severe high blood pressure which should be prescribed during hospitalization.

It is one of the few drugs that can be used during pregnancy.

Common Vasodilator Drugs:
- Minoxidil
- Hydralazine

Side-effects of Vasodilators:
- Headache, flushing and palpitations are frequent side-effects of vasodilators.
- Vasodilators, when used alone, may worsen angina.
- Ankle swelling is another side-effect and is due to the retention of salt and water by the kidneys; a diuretic may counteract this.
- In high doses, about 200 mg or more per day, hydralazine may induce an autoimmune disease called lupus erythematous (LE) in about one third of the people who take it and in 1–3% of people even below this dose. This happens more commonly in

women than men. In this disease, patient produces antibodies against his own body, resulting in painful swollen joints. LE usually starts as widespread joint pains and swelling, closely resembles rheumatoid arthritis. Unless the possibility of LE is kept in mind. It is imagined that patient has developed another disorder and to start treating the consequences instead of the cause.

- Minoxidil may increase hair growth on the body, giving women hair growth but causing some regrowth in bald men.
- In rare cases, minoxidil may cause accumulation of water in the pericardium (covering of the heart). This side-effect is reversible.

Group 6: Alpha-blocker

They reduce blood pressure by dilating (widening) the small arteries. These work by blocking the action of the hormone adrenaline on muscles that make up the walls of blood vessels. Adrenaline make the blood vessel constrict. Blocking these receptors make the blood vessels relax and dilating, and blood pressure falls.

Individual response to these drugs varies a lot, so treatment should be started with a small dose and slowly increased. Once the right dose has been found, they are generally trouble free for most people until they reach their late 70s.

They seem to be safe in pregnancy. Alpha-blockers reduce blood cholesterol significantly. This cholesterol lowering effect is an important advantage.

Alpha-blockers have other functions as well as controlling blood pressure. They have been shown, particularly to relax the bladder so that they improve the flow of urine in males with moderate obstruction from benign enlargement of the prostate. This is extremely common in late middle-age and usage of alpha-blockers postpone the surgery.

Common Alpha-blockers:
- Prazosin
- Doxazosin
- Terzosin
- Indoramin
- Phentolamin mesylate
- Phenoxybenzamine hydrochloride

Side effect of Alpha-blockers:
- Alpha-blockers can cause dizziness, especially when someone stand up suddenly, unless it is given last thing at night before going to bed. Doxazosin and terazonsin may still cause some dizziness in some individual. Fainting is a problem in elderly people even after the use of these drug is well established. Alpha-blockers should not therefore be used for the people of old age.
- They can cause light-headedness and a dry mouth
- They may occasionally cause some stress and incontinence among women. This is reversible once the tablets are stopped.

Group 7: Calcium Channel Blockers

Calcium channel blockers (also known as calcium antagonists) work by blocking the transfer of calcium ions across cell membrane in the smooth muscle of the wall of the arterioles, mainly in the heart. It is thought that constriction of the smooth muscle caused by calcium, narrow these blood vessels, which causes rise in blood pressure. Blocking the action of calcium open up the blood vessels and results in a fall in blood pressure.

However, they have no effect on calcium of bones and no effect on osteoporosis. They are also effective in controlling angina.

Verapamil (Cordilox, Securon) has a large effect on the heart and was originally recommended only for control of arrhythmias (abnormal heart rhythms). It can be dangerous if combined with beta-blockers, because this combination may precipitate heart failure or dangerous disturbances in heart rhythm. Dittiazem (Adizem, Tildiem) is particularly effective for some people with beta-blockers. All the other drugs of this group are all effective and well tolerated even in combination with beta-blockers. They are particularly effective in older people.

Common Calcium Channel Blockers:

- Diltiazem hydrochloride
- Nicardipine hydrochloride
- Verapamil hydrochloride
- Lercanidipine hydrochloride
- Amlodipine besylate
- Nifedipine
- Felodipline
- Lacidipine
- Nisolaipine
- Isradipine

Side-effects of Calcium Channel Blockers:

- The problem is that all arterioles open up, including the brain, which can lead to headaches; the face, which can cause flushing; and in legs, which can result in ankle swelling, particularly the formulation produces fewer effects. Amlodipine and lacidipine cause few problems, high doses do cause ankle swelling. These side-effects are much less common with slow-release (SR) preparations.

- Verapamil can cause constipation and may also be hazardous in certain form of heart disease

- Calcium channel blockers should be avoided in pregnancy, as they may delay the start of labour and some drugs in this group have caused fetal deformities

Group 8: Drugs Acting Mainly on Brainstem

These drug work by action on the brainstem (lies between brain and spinal cord) that controls blood pressure. The brainstem controls many automatic bodily functions, including heart output, the diameter of small arteries in different parts of the body and urine output.

Newer drugs have fewer side effects and are equally safe, so methyldopa is now usually used only when other drugs have been found to be ineffective in reducing blood pressure.

Methyldopa remains very popular for treatment of high blood pressure during pregnancy. There is good evidence that methyldopa is safe in pregnancy and there will be no adverse effects on the development of baby.

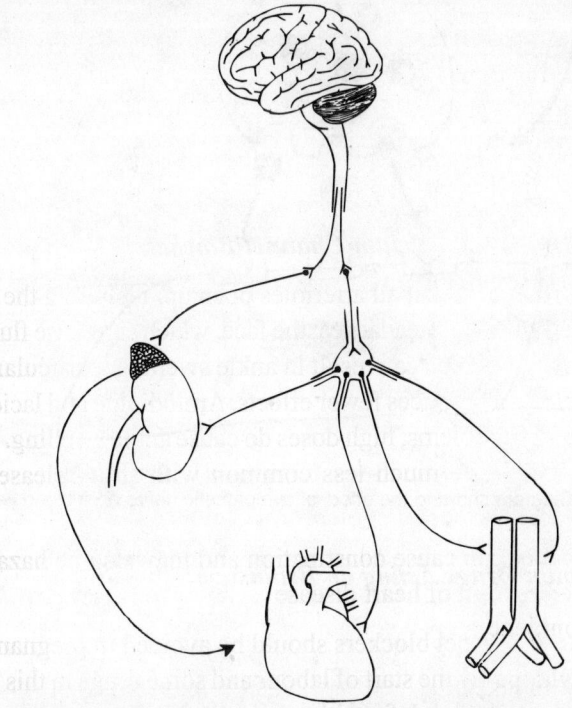

Fig. 27: Diagramatic representation of the sympathetic nervous system

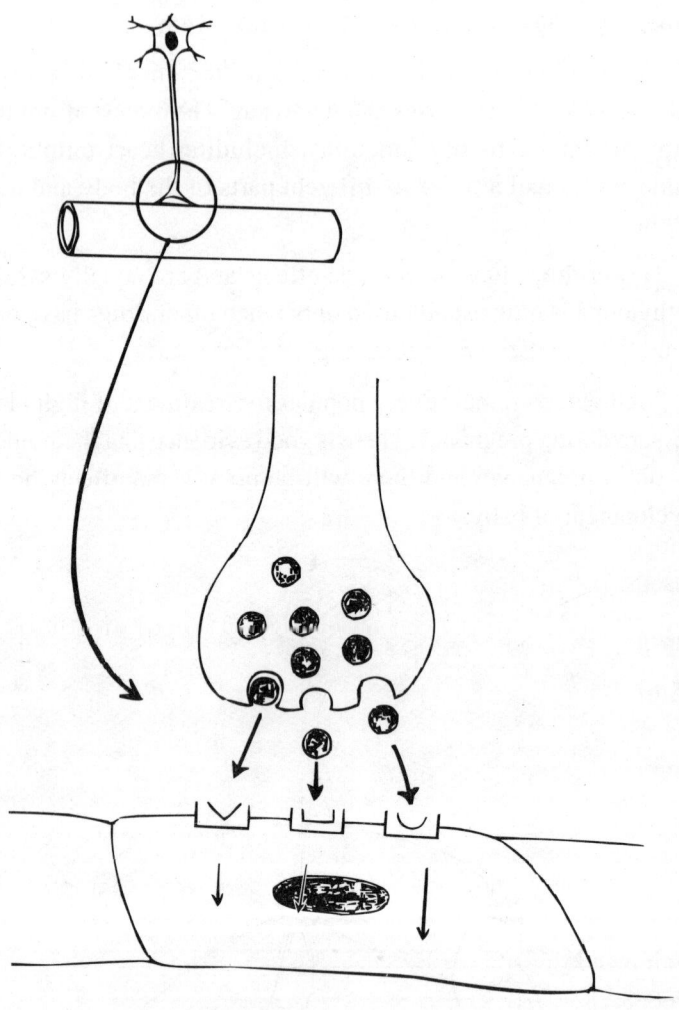

Fig. 28: Diagram showing the effect of sympathetic nerve on a blood vessel

Common Drugs Acting on Brainstem:

- Moxonidene
- Methyldopa
- Clonidine hydrochloride

Side-effects of Drugs Acting on Brainstem:

- They do tend to cause tiredness, lethargy, drowsiness, dreams, depression, stuffy nose and dry mouth, particularly in high doses. None should be used by people already prone to experience depression.

- Methyldopa can cause liver damage, particularly in elderly people and sometimes severe enough to cause jaundice. Blood tests in this condition resemble the test results of infectious jaundice, gall stones or toxic effects of some drugs.

- They can also cause impotency which is reversible when the drug is stopped.

- Clonidine can cause dangerous high blood pressure if it is stopped suddenly (rebound blood pressure), so it can only be used safely in a slow release (SR) form.

Group 9: Adrenergic Neuron Blockers

Adrenergic neuron blockers were first introduced in 1959. These drugs are now very rarely used and used only during hospitalization.

Side-effects of Adrenergic Neuron Blockers:

- All of these drugs tend to cause troublesome diarrhea and delayed or impaired ejaculation

- Fainting is main side-effect of adrenergic neuron blockers. People need to avoid rapid head movements, need to climb up and descends stairs slowly, use a stick for support when walking and avoid heights.

Group 10: Ganglion Blockers

Ganglion blockers work by blocking the nerves that control the spiral muscles around the small arteries, so increases their diameter. They are like adrenergic neuron blockers used only rarely and only during hospitalization.

Side-effects of Ganglion Blockers:

- They may cause flushing because the effects are wide-spread rather than concentrated on target arteries and the fall in pressure is usually large
- These drugs tend to increase heart rate

Table: Showing Different Brand Names of Drugs

Group No.	Generic Name	Brand Name
IA	Bendofluazide	Aprinox, Prestim, Presmtim forte, Noe-Naclex, Corgaretic 40, Corgaretic 80, Inderetic
IA	Benzthiazide	Dytide
IA	Chlorthalidone	Hygroton, Kalspare, Tenoret 50, Tenoretic
IA	Chlorothiazide	Saluric
IA	Clopamide	Viskaldix
IA	Cyclopenthiazide	Navidrex, Navispare, Trasidrex
IA	Hydrochorothiazide	Amil-co, Capozide, Dynazide, Kalten, Hydro Saluric, Acezide, Accuretic Capozidels, Traim-co, Moducren, Innozide Moduret 25, Moduretic, Carace 10 plus, Carace 20 plus, Co-Betoloc cozaar-comp, Monozide 10, Secudrex, Zestoretic
IA	Hydroflumethiazide	Aldactide
IA	Indapamide	Natrilix, Natrilix SR, Natramid
IA	Mefruside	Baycaron
IA	Metolazone	Metenix 5
IA	Polythiazide	Nephril
IA	Xipamide	Diurexan
IB	Amiloride	Amil-co, Navispare, Frumil, Burinex A, Moducren, Moduretic, Moduret, Kalten
IB	Triameterene	Kalspare, Dyazide, Frusene, Train-co.

Group No.	Generic Name	Brand Name
1C	Potassium Chloride	Neo-Naclex-K, Burinex-K, Continus, Lasikal, Lasix-K, Diumide-K
1D	Bumetanide	Burinex-A, Burinex, Burinex-K
1D	Ethacrynic acid	Edecrin
1D	Torasemide	Torem
2	Acebutolol	Sectral, Secadrex
2	Atenolol	Tomato, Beta-Adalat, Tenormin, Tenoretic, Tenif, Kalten, Tenoret 50, Tenormin-LS
2	Betaxolol	Kerlone
2	Bisoprolol	Eucardic
2	Celiprolol	Celectrol
2	labetalol	Trandate
2	Metoprolol	Lopresor, Lopresor, Sr, Betaloc, Co-Betaloc
2	Nadolol	Corgard, Corgaretic
2	Oxprenolol	Trasicor, Slow-Trasicor, Trasidrex
2	Pindolol	Visken, Viskaldix
2	Propranolol	Inderex, Inderal, Half-Inderals, Inderetic, Beta-Progran,e Probeta LA
2	Sotalol	Beta-Cardone
2	Timolol	Prestim Forte, Prestim, Betim, Moducren, Blocardren
3	Captopril	Capoten, Capozide, Capozide LS, Acepril, Acezide
3	Cilazapril	Vascace
3	Enalapril	Innozide, Innovace
3	Fosinopril	Staril
3	Lisnopril	Zestril, Carace, Carace 10 plus, Zestoretic
3	Mexipril	Perdix
3	Perindopril	Coversyl
3	Quinapril	Aceuretic, Accupro

Group No.	Generic Name	Brand Name
3	Ramipril	Tritace
3	Trandolapril	Odrik, Gopten
4	Cendasartan	Amias
4	Irbesartan	Aprovel
4	Valsartan	Diovan
5	Hydralazine	Apresoline
5	Minoxidil	Loniten
6	Doxazosin	Cardura
6	Indoramin	Doralese, Baratol
6	Prazosin	Hypavase
6	Terazosin	Hytrin
7	Amoldipin	Istin
7	Diltiazem	Dilzem-SR, Slozem, Adizem, Adizem-SR, Adizem-XL, Tildiem-LA, Tildiem Retard, Angitil-SR
7	Felodipin	Plendil
7	Isradipine	Prescal
7.	Lacidipine	Motens
7	Larcanidipine	Zanidip
7	Nicardipine	Cardene, Cardene-SR
7	Nifedipine	Angiopine-MR, Calanif, Tenif, Adalat Retard, Beta-Adalat, Calanif, Cardilate-MR, Adalat-LA, Tensipine, Nifensar-XL, Coracten, Unipine
7	Nisoldripine	Syscor-MR
7	Verapamil	Securon, Securon-SR, Univer, Cordilox, Half-Securon-SR
8	Clonidipne	Catapres, Catapres, Perlongets
8	Methyldoph	Aldomet
8	Moxonidine	Physiotens
9	Bethanidine	Bendoger
9	Debrisoquire	—
9	Guanethidine	Ismelin

Combination Therapy

It is considered best to use two or more blood pressure-lowering drugs in lower doses rather than any one drug in a high dose. About half of the people with high blood pressure need to take more than one drug to control it, but this would only mean taking a maximum of four tablets sometimes fewer in a day. All drugs can be taken together once daily so even quadruple therapy requires only four gills a unit of liquid measure, equal to a quater of a pint taken together.

Certain combination of drugs are more effective than others. In general the beta-blockers and ACE inhibitors are best given with either thiazide diuretics or calcium channel blockers. There is often not much to be gained by combining a beta-blockers with an ACE-inhibitors or combining a thiazide diuretics with a calcium channel blockers.

Monitoring and Follow-up

Before anyone starts on treatment for high blood pressure several measurements need to be made on different days at least on three or often more. The reason, high blood pressure needs treatment is to reduce the risks of suffering from coronary heart disease, stroke or any other complications, eventually.

Drugs used for treatment of high blood pressure often cause side effects. It is important to report these to doctor, because they can always be avoided by changing the drug or changing the dose. Angina (pain over the front of the chest on exertion) and claudication (leg pain from obstructed leg arteries) are increasingly common in men from middle age onwards, and are much more likely in people with high blood pressure, even if this has been controlled by treatment. Both these complaints should be reported to doctor.

About 20 to 30% of people treated for high blood pressure are unable to respond to the drugs. The commonest causes of failure to respond to drugs are:

- A high alcohol intake
- Taking ACE-inhibitors drug without reducing amount of salt in the diet
- Severe depression
- People forgetting to take their tablets, but being too afraid to admit this

If all these causes are excluded, the next possibility is rare cause of secondary high blood pressure, which will need investigations.

Physician is doing follow-up will check all these things:

- How much one smoke
- Weight for height
- Regular exercise habits
- Blood cholesterol level

About once in every year, person should also have urine test and a blood test to check his protein urea and creatinine levels. A test for glucose is important because diabetes is a common complications of high blood pressure. Patient with diabetes, need to have a routine examination of their retina once a year but if blood pressure is under control and diabetes is absent then this is not necessary.

Chapter 12

Homeopathic Treatment

1. Rauwolfia Serpentina (Serpagandha)

Symptoms

- Its main sphere of action is high blood pressure
- *Irritable condition of the central nervous system*
- In high blood pressure without marked changes in the vessels
- Insanity, violent maniacal symptoms
- It helps in sleeping

Doses: Rauwolfia Serpentia ϕ, 10–15 drops three times daily for one month.

2. Crataegus (Hawthorn Berries)

Symptoms

- It is a *heart tonic*. It acts on muscles of heart
- Reduces blood pressure
- Chronic heart disease with extreme weakness
- Produces giddiness and lowered pulse

- *Extreme difficult respiration on least exertion*, without much increase of pulse
- Cardiac dropsy
- Very feeble and irregular heart action
- Pain in the region of *heart and under left ventricle*
- *Arteriosclerosis* said to have a solvent power upon crustaceous and calcareous deposits in arteries
- Heart muscles seem flabby and worn out
- Difficulty in breathing and nervous prostration, with heart failure
- Pulse accelerated, *irregular, feeble and intermittent*
- *Heart dilated and first sound weak*
- Angina pectoris
- Anaemia, oedema
- Cutaneous chilliness, blueness of fingers and toes, aggravated by exertion or excitement
- Cold extremities, pallor, irregular pulse and breathing
- Very nervous and irritable with pain in back of head and neck
- Insomnia of aortic patient
- *Diabetes*, especially in children
- Excessive perspiration. Skin eruptions

Symptoms Worse

- In warm room

Symptoms Better

- Fresh air, quiet and rest

Doses: Crataegus φ, 15 drops in water three times daily for 3 months.

3. Natrum Muriaticum (Common Salt)

Symptoms

- A great remedy for certain forms of intermittent fever anaemia whether from loss of vital fluids; profuse menses, seminal losses—or mental affections
- Heart and chest feel constricted
- Increased heart beat rate
- Fluttering, palpitation, intermittent pulse. *Intermits on lying down*
- Heart pulsation shake body
- Great debility; most weakness felt in the morning in bed
- Great liability to take cold
- **Great emaciation; losing flesh while living well; great weakness and weariness**
- Irritable, disposition to weep; without cause, *but consolation aggravates*
- Ill effects of shock, grief anger, fright, resentment or humiliation
- *Dreams of robbers* in the house.
- Thirst for cold drinks throughout.
- Craving for salts and aversion to bread
- For the bad effects of acid food, bread, quinine, excessive use of salts; of cauterization of all kinds with the silver nitrate

Symptoms *Worse*

- 10 to 11 a.m.
- At seashore or from sea air.
- On lying down especially of left side.
- Heat of sun or fire.
- From noise, music.
- From mental exertion.
- Consolation.
- Talking, writing, reading.

Symptoms *Better*

- In the open air.
- By sweat.
- From cold bathing.
- Going *without regular meals* (while fasting).
- Pressure against back.
- Lying on right side.
- Tight clothing.

- *Sweats while eating*
- Heartburn, with palpitation
- Headache—as if a thousand little hammers were knocking on the brain, in the morning on awakening, *before or after menstruation*, by bright sunlight, or by severe coughing, *from sunrise to sunset*
- Headache: anaemia, of school girls
- Chronic headache, semi-lateral, congestive with pale face, nausea and vomiting, periodical in nature, from eyestrain
- Headache better from rest, sweating
- *Eye muscles weak and stiff*
- Eye feel bruised with headaches in school children
- *Tears stream down the face whenever he coughs*
- Pain in eyes when looking down
- *Violent, fluent coryza*. Discharge thin and watery like raw white of egg
- *Loss of smell and taste*
- Numbness, tingling of tongue, lips and nose
- Tongue *mapped, with red insular patches*, heavy, difficult speech, children slow in learning to walk
- Lips and corner of mouth dry, ulcerated and cracked
- Pain just after urination. Has to wait a long time for it to pass if other are present. Urine involuntary when walking, coughing, laughing.
- Constipation, stool dry hard, difficult, crumbling; anus constricted, torn, bleeding
- Cough with bursting pain in head. Whooping-cough with flow of tears with cough.

- Numbness and tingling in finger and lower extremities
- Crackling in joints on motion
- Pain in back with desire for some firm support
- Palms hot and perspiring
- Dryness and cracking about fingernails. Hang nails.
- Dry eruptions, especially on margin of hairy scalp and bands of joints
- Eczema, *crusty eruptions in bend of limbs, margin of scalp,* behind ears worse at seashore.

Doses: Natrium muriaticum 30, 4 pills three times daily for one month.

4. Glonoine (Nitro-glycerine)

Symptoms

- Great remedy for congestive headaches, hyperemia of the brain from excess of heat or cold
- *Surging of blood to head and heart*
- Tendency to sudden and violent irregularities of the circulation
- *Sensation of pulsation throughout the body.* Pulsating pains.
- Violent pulsation with difficult breathing cannot go uphill
- Hearts action labored, oppressed; blood seems to rush to heart and rapidly to head
- Any exertion brings on rush of blood to heart and fainting spells
- Throbbing in the whole body to fingertips
- *Head heavy but cannot lay it on pillow cannot bear any heat about head*
- Throbbing headache, holds head with both hands

- Head feels enormously large, as if skull were too small for brain, blood seems to be pumping upward; throbs at every jar, step, pulse
- **Sun stroke and sun headache**; increases and decreases everyday with the sun
- **Headache in place of menses**
- Vertigo on assuming upright position
- *Confusion* with dizziness
- Head trouble from working under gaslight, when heat falls on head, heat of stove or walking in the sun and from having the hair cut
- Children get sick in the evening when sitting before an open fire or falling asleep there
- Headache better from cool air, lying down, sleep, head held high
- Headache occurring after profuse uterine hemorrhage, rush of blood to head, in pregnant women
- Flushes of heat in women, at menses or in pregnancy or at the climacterics
- Bad effects of mental excitement, fright fear, mechanical injuries and their later consequences, from having the hair cut
- Neck feels full. Collars must be opened.
- Nausea and vomiting of cerebral origin. Faint, gnawing and empty feeling at pit of stomach.
- Painful piles with pinching in abdomen before and after stool

Symptoms Worse

- In the sun, exposure to sun's rays
- Gas-light
- Over heating
- Having hair-cut
- Stooping
- Jar
- Ascending
- Peaches
- Stimulants
- Lying down
- From 6 a.m. to noon

Symptoms Better

- In open air
- From cold
- From brandy
- From pressure

- Drawing pain in all limbs. Backache.
- Convulsion and meningitis in children

    Doses: Glonoine 30, 4 pills three times daily for one month

5. Viscum Album (Mistletoe)

Symptoms

- It lowers blood pressure
- Pulse small and weak
- Hypertrophy of heart with valvular insufficiency
- Palpitation during coitus
- Difficult breathing worse lying on left side
- Weight and oppression of heart, as if a hand were squeezing it
- Tickling sensation about heart
- Systolic pressure high and diastolic low
- Patient unable to rest in a reclining position
- Albumin in urine in high blood pressure patient
- Mainly affects rheumatic any gouty complaints, neuralgia especially *sciatica*
- Rheumatism with tearing pains
- *Tearing*, shooting pain in both thighs and upper extremities
- Pain alternate in the knee and ankle with shoulder and elbow respectively
- Periodic pains from sacrum into pelvis, *worse in bed*, with pains into thighs and upper extremities
- *Rheumatic deafness*. Buzzing and stopped-up feeling in ear

Symptoms Worse
- Cold, stormy weather
- Winter
- Lying on left side
- In bed
- Movement

- *Asthma,* if connected with gout or rheumatism
- *Difficult breathing, feeling suffocation when lying on left side*
- Blue ring around eyes
- Uterine hemorrhage in female, with pain, blood partly clotted and bright red
- Climacteric complaints in females
- Epilepsy and chorea

Dose: Viscum album ϕ, 15 drops in water, two times daily, for one month.

6. Aurum Metallicum (Metallic Gold)

Symptoms

- It generally affect the blood, glands and bone
- *High blood pressure*, night paroxysms of pain behind sternum
- *Arteriosclerosis*; palpitation and congestion
- *Sensation as if heart stopped beating* for two or three seconds, immediately followed by a tumultuous rebound, with sinking at the epigastrium
- Violent palpitation, anxiety with congestion of blood to heart and chest after exertion
- Pulse *small, feeble, rapid, irregular*, visible beating of carotid and temporal arteries
- Fatty degeneration of heart
- For constitution broken down by bad effects of mercury and syphilis
- Hopeless, despondent, depressed and **great desire to commit suicide**

- Profound despondency, with increased blood pressure, *with thorough disgust of life* and thoughts of suicide
- *Talks of committing suicide*
- Ailments from fright, anger, contradiction, mortification, vexation, dread
- **Profound melancholy**; feels hateful and quarrelsome, desire to commit suicide, life is constant burden
- *Oversensitive*; to noise, excitement, to smell, taste, hearing, touch, to pain, least contradiction excites wrath
- Uneasy, hurried, great desire for mental and physical activity; cannot do things fast enough. Constant rapid questioning without waiting for reply.
- *Voilent pressure in head, worse at night*
- Falling of the hair, especially in syphilis and mercurial affections
- *Extreme photophobia. Upper half of objects invisible* sees only the lower half.
- Carries of the nasal palatine and mastoid bones; obstinate fetid otorrhoea, ozena pain worse at night
- *Pain and swelling of testicles*, chronic induration of testicles.
- Atrophy of testicles in boys
- Prolapse and indurated uterus; from over—reaching or strain, from hypertrophy
- Pain in bones of head, lumps under scalp, exostosis with nightly pains in bones

Symptoms Worse

- In cold weather when getting cold
- Many complaints come on only in winter
- While lying down
- Mental exertion
- From sunset to sunrise

Symptoms Better

- In warm air
- When growing warm
- During summer
- In the morning

- All the blood seems to rush from head to lower limbs

Dose: Aurum metallicum 30, 4 pills three times daily for one month.

7. Cactus Grandiflorus (Night—Blooming Cereus)

Symptoms

- Acts on circular muscular fibres, hence create constriction, especially on heart and arteries, producing very characteristic *constrictions* as of an iron hand
- Atheromatous arteries and weak heart
- *Favors speedy clot formation*
- Angina pectoris with suffocation, cold sweat and ever present iron-band feeling
- Pain in apex (left side of chest) shooting down left arm
- *Endocarditis with mitral insufficiency together with violent and rapid action*
- Congestion, irregular distribution of blood
- Endocardial murmurs, excessive impulse, increased precordial dullness, enlarged ventricle
- Violent palpitation day and night *worse lying of left* side, at *approach of menses* and *walking*
- Palpitation with vertigo, difficult breathing and flatulence
- *Constriction*, very acute pains and stitches in heart, pulse feeble, irregular, quick, without strength

Symptoms *Worse*
• Lying *on left side*
• About noon
• 11 a.m. and 11 p.m
• Walking
• Going upstairs

Symptoms *Better*
• Open air

- Heart feels as if *clasped and unclasped rapidly by* an *iron band,* as if bound; had no room to beat
- Low blood pressure
- *Constriction in chest as if bound, hindering respiration*
- Oppressed breathing as from a weight on chest
- *Heart-constriction as from an iron hand*
- Inflammation of diaphragm, with great difficulty of breathing
- **Hemorrhage, constrictions, periodicity and spasmodic pains** are characteristics of this remedy
- Hemorrhage: From nose, lungs, stomach, rectum and bladder
- **Whole** body **feels as if caged**, each wire being twisted tighter and tighter
- Pain everywhere; darting, spasmodic and ending with a sharp, vice-like grip, only to be again renewed
- **Constriction**: Of throat, chest, heart, bladder, rectum vagina; often caused or brought on by the slightest contact sensation as of a weight on vertex
- Right-sided headache and neuralgia; congestive, pulsating and periodical headache
- Dryness of tongue, as if burnt, needs much liquid to get food down
- Toxic goiter with cardiac symptoms
- *Painful menses*, pulsating pain in uterus and ovaries
- Menses early, dark, pitch-like, *cease on lying down*, with heart symptoms
- Edema of hands and feet
- Numbness of left arm

- Fever every day at same hour, paroxysms, about 11 a.m. and 11 p.m., accompanied by hemorrhages. Coldness predominates, icy-cold hands, cold sweat.

Dose: Cactus grandiflorus ϕ, 15 drops in water, twice daily for one month.

8. Baryta Muriatica (Barium Chloride)

Symptoms

- Arteriosclerosis and cerebral affections are caused by this remedy
- High blood pressure and vascular degeneration
- Arteriosclerosis where a high systolic pressure with a comparatively low diastolic tension with cardiac and cerebral symptoms
- Increased tension of pulse
- The white blood cells increased
- Headache occurring in old people, heaviness rather than pain
- Voices, due to anaemia and noises in ears
- Chronic hypertrophy of the tonsils, children who go around with their mouth open and who talk through the nose
- Parotids swollen, offensive otorrhoea
- *Narrowing of the cardiac orifice with pain,* immediately after eating and epigastric tenderness
- *All gone feeling at epigastrium*
- *Induration of pancreas and* spasmodic pain in rectum
- *Bronchial affections of old people* with *cardiac dilation. Facilitates expectoration* and rattling of mucus with difficult expectoration.

- *Icy coldness of body with paralysis*
- Voluntary muscular power gone but perfectly sensible
- General feeling of lassitude in the morning, specially weakness of legs, with muscular stiffness
- Great increase in uric-acid

    Dose: Baryta muriatica 30, 4 pills thrice daily for one month.

9. Boerhaavia Diffusa (Punarnaba)

Symptoms

- Acts on high blood pressure and heart troubles
- It also acts on asthma, beri-beri, dropsy, jaundice, gonorrhoea
- Terrible, bursting, right sided headache better by cold applications
- Giddiness present
- Frequent palpitation and intermittent throbbing pain in cardiac region
- Swelling of eye lids, hands, abdomen, legs and feet
- Scanty, high colored urine
- *Coryza, with dry cough* and thick white expectoration
- Rheumatic pain all over body
- Slight *pain in the hepatic region* was felt on touch or pressure and better by hard pressure
- Sleeplessness with heaviness in head
- Cirrhosis of liver
- *Symptoms get worse* when alone

    Doses: Boerhaavia Diffusa φ, drops in water thrice daily.

10. Gelsemium Sempevirens (Yellow Jasmine)

Symptoms

- It acts mainly upon the nervous system
- *Dizziness, dullness, drowsiness, and trembling* is the main characteristic of the medicine
- For children, young people, especially women of a nervous hysterical temperament
- Excitable, irritable and sensitive person
- Bad effects from fright, fear, exciting news and sudden emotions
- Desire to be quite, to be left alone; does not wish to speak or have any one near her, even if the person be silent
- *Apathy regarding his illness*
- Stage fright, nervous dread of appearing in public; the anticipation of any unusual ordeal preparing for theatre, church or to meet an engagement, brings on diarrhoea
- *A feeling as if it were necessary* to keep *in motion*, or *else heart's action would cease*
- Pulse slow when quiet, but greatly accelerated on motion
- *Weak, slow pulse of old age*
- Palpitation; pulse soft, weak, fall and flowing

Symptoms Worse
• Damp weather
• Before a thunderstorm
• Emotion or excitement
• Bad news
• When thinking of his ailments
• Tobacco smoking
• At 10 a.m.

Symptoms Better
• Bending forward
• By profuse urination
• Continued motion
• Open air
• Stimulants

- Heaviness of head *band-feeling around* and occipital headache
- *Pain in temple, extending into ear* and wing of nose, causing a bursting sensation in forehead and eye
- Dull, heavy headache with heaviness of eye lids, better compression and lying with head high
- Headache preceded by blindness; better by profuse urination
- *Vertigo*, spreading from occiput, with dim vision, loss of vision, seems intoxicated when trying to move
- General depression *from heat of sun or summer*
- *Muscular weakness and trembling*; of tongue, hands, legs and of the entire body
- Great heaviness of eyelids, cannot keep them open
- *Orbital neuralgia*, with contraction and twitching of muscles of eyes
- Hot, heavy, flushed, besotted-looking face
- Feeling of a lump in throat that cannot be swallowed
- *Pain from throat to ear*
- *Retention* of urine. Profuse, clear, watery urine.
- *Lack of muscular coordinations*; confused; muscles refuse to obey the will
- Complete relaxation and prostration of the whole muscular system with motor paralysis
- Fever with nervous chill without thirst, especially along the spine, running up and down the back in rapid, wave-like succession from sacrum occiput
- *Measles, catarrhal symptoms*. Aids in bringing out eruption.

Dose: Gelsemium 30, 4 pills thrice daily for one month

11. Uranium Nitricum (Nitrate of Uranium)

Symptoms

- It is known to produce diabetes, degeneration of the liver, high blood pressure, nephritis and dropsy
- Therapeutic keynote of Uranium nitricum is *debility, great emaciation and tendency to ascites and general dropsy*
- It causes increased frequency of urine and glycosuria
- Incontinence of urine
- *Burning in urethra*, with very acid urine
- Unable to retain urine without pain
- Dull, heavy pain in head
- Mental depression
- High blood pressure during dropsy
- Styes with lids inflamed and agglutinated
- Nausea, *vomiting* and excessive thirst
- *Gastric and duodenal ulcers*, burning pain in abdomen
- *Ravenous appetite* eating followed by flatulence. *Abdomen bloated* due to gas.
- Burning pain in pyloric region
- Complete impotency, with nocturnal emissions

Doses: Uranium nitricum 3X, 4 pills four times daily for one month.

12. Conium Maculatum (Poison Hemlock)

Symptoms

- Great debility in the morning in bed. *Weakness of body and mind, trembling* and palpitation

- Cancerous diathesis
- High blood pressure of bachelors and maids in old age
- *Anxious, depressed memory* weak sensitive to noise
- Insomnia, before midnight and with nightmares
- *Vertigo, when lying down and when turning over in bed*, when turning head sidewise
- Headache with nausea and vomiting of mucus. Tightness as if both temples were compressed, *worse after a meal.*
- *Enlarged glands.* Act on the glandular system, engorging and indurating it.
- *Axillary gland pain, with numb* feeling down the arm
- *Breast enlarged and become painful* before and during menses. Wants to press breast hard with hand.
- Breast lumps worse in right breast
- Photophobia and excessive lachrymation
- Conium is a excellent remedy for difficult gait, trembling, sudden loss of strength while walking, painful stiffness of legs
- *Muscular weakness,* especially of lower extremities. *Putting feet on chair relieves pain*
- Ascending paralysis, ending in death by failure of respiration.
- Perspiration of hands
- Terrible nausea, acrid heartburn, worse on going to bed.

Symptoms Worse
- On lying down
- Turning or rising in bed
- Bodily or mental exertion
- Before and during menses
- From taking cold

Symptoms Better
- From sitting down
- From letting limbs hang down
- While fasting
- From pressure
- In the dark

- Amelioration from eating and aggravation a few hours after meals.
- Frequent urging for stool. *Tremulous weakness after every stool.*
- *Interrupted discharge of urine.* It flows and stops again.
- Dry, irritating, tickling, violent cough worse evening and night, when lying down; must sit up as soon as cough starts. Expectoration difficult.

Dose: Conium mac 30, 4 pills thrice daily for one month.

13. Calearea Carbonica (Carbonate of Lime)

Symptoms

- The keynote action of this remedy is on the glands, skin and bones
- Psoric constitution, pale, weak, easily tired
- Persons of scrofulous type, who take cold easily
- Leucophlegmatic temperament, light complexion, pale skin, large head, blue eyes; tendency to grow fat in children
- Calcarea patient is fair, fat, flabby and perspiring and cold
- Disposed to grow fat
- Children with large heads and abdomens; fontanelles and sutures open, bones soft, develop very slowly difficult and delayed dentition; who takes *cold easily* and sweat easily
- *Girls who are fleshy, plethoric and grow too rapidly*
- *Apprehensive, forgetful* and confused
- Fear of loss of reason
- Vertigo on ascending and when turning head
- **Head sweats profusely while sleeping, wetting pillow**

- Profuse perspiration, mostly on back of head and neck or chest or upper part of body. Sweat of single parts.
- Longing for fresh air, when in a room
- *Great liability to take cold*
- Coldness of single part; head, stomach, abdomen, feet and legs, especially right side
- *Craving for indigestible thing like chalk, coal, great longing for eggs.* Aversion to meat.
- Diseases arising from defective assimilation; imperfect ossification; difficulty in learning to walk or stand. It is indicated in children have no disposition to walk and will not try
- *Frequent sour eructation, sour vomiting. Loss of appetite when overworked.*
- Pit of stomach swollen like an *inverted saucer* and painful to pressure
- Feels better in every way when constipated. Stool needs to be removed mechanically. Stool at first hard, then pasty and then liquid.
- All discharges, e.g. sweat, diarrhea and vomiting smell sour
- Tendency of developing polyps in nose
- *Swelling of tonsils* and sub-maxillary gland
- Amenorrhea caused by working in water

Symptoms Worse

- In cold wet weather
- Cold air
- Cold in every form; water, washing, moist air
- During full moon
- Morning
- From exertion, mental or physical
- Ascending

Symptoms Better

- Dry weather
- Lying on painful side
- From rubbing
- Sneezing (pain in head and nape)
- From drawing the limbs up

- Menses *too early, too profuse, too long* with vertigo, tootache; feet habitually cold and damp, as if they had on cold damp stockings
- The least mental excitement causes profuse return of menstrual flow
- Leucorrhea, thick milky discharge during maturation or flowing only in spells. Discharge is acrid, corroding the genitals.
- Extreme dyspnoea
- *Painless hoarseness*, worse in the morning
- *Suffocative spells,* tightness, burning and soreness in chest, *worse going upstairs* or slightest ascent, must sit down
- *Chest very sensitive to touch, percussion or pressure*
- Palpitation at night and after eating
- Rheumatic and gouty conditions of joints, swelling of joints, especially knees
- *Rawness of soles of feet*, blisters and offensive foot sweat
- Frequent waking at night. Some disagreeable idea always arouse him from light slumber.

Dose: Calcarea carbonica 30, 4 pills thrice daily for 15 days. It should not be repeated too frequently in old people.

14. Passiflora Incarnata (Passion-flower)

Symptoms

- Has a quietening effect on the nervous system
- In insomnia, produces normal sleep
- Insomina of infants and the aged, and the mentally worried, and overworked, with tendency to convulsions
- Restless and wakeful sleep, resulting from exhaustion

- Violent headache as if top of head would come of—eyes felt as it pushed out
- An efficient *antispasmodic*
- Used in cases whooping-cough
- *Asthma* with nocturnal cough
- Delirium tremens, convulsions in children, neuralgia
- Neuroses of children, worm-fever, teething spasms
- *Tetanus*
- Painful diarrhea
- Laden, dead feeling after or between meals; flatulence and sour eructations

Dose: Passiflora incarnata φ, 10 drops in water, thrice daily for one month.

15. Baryta Carbonica (Carbonate of Baryta)

Symptoms

- It especially suits to complaints of first and second childhood (extremes of life) i.e. infants and old people
- Person subject to quinsy, *take cold easily*, even the least cold precipitates an attack of tonsillitis, prone to suppuration
- It brings aid to scrofulous, dwarfish children who do not grow and develop, swollen abdomen, face bloated, general emaciation, take cold easily and *then always have swollen tonsils*
- *Children both physically and mentally weak*
- Difficulty in learning at school; bad memory of children, cannot concentrate
- *Disease of old men,* with physical and mental weakness, when degenerative changes begin—cardiovascular and cerebral;

hypertrophy or induration of prostate, very sensitive to take cold, offensive foot sweats, childishness; thoughtless behavior

- Often useful in the dyspepsia of the young who suffer from seminal emissions, together with cardiac irritability and palpitation

- Baryta is a cardiovascular poison acting on the muscular coats of heart and vessels

- Arterial fibrosis. Blood vessels soften and degenerate, become distended and aneurysms.

- Accelerates the hearts' action. At first, blood pressure much increased and contraction of blood-vessels.

- Palpitation and distress in region of heart

- Palpitation when lying of left side, pulse full and hard

- Cardiac symptoms after suppressed foot-sweat

- Apoplectic tendency in old people; complaints of old drunkards; headache of aged people, who are childish

- Swelling and indurations, or incipient suppuration of glands, specially cervical and inguinal.

- Offensive foot sweats, toes and soles get sore

- Glands around ears painful and swollen. Crackling noise in the ear.

- Sub-maxillary glands and tonsils swollen

- Take cold easily, with stitching and smarting pain in throat

Symptoms Worse

- While thinking of complaints
- Lying on painful side
- From washing
- After meals
- In the morning
- While sitting

Symptoms Better

- Walking in open air
- When standing
- From motion

- Suppurating tonsils form every cold
- Inability to swallow anything but liquids
- Throat affections after checked foot sweat
- Hard and tense, distended abdomen with pain in abdomen
- Dwarfish, hysterical women and old maids with scanty menses, deficient heart, always cold and chilly
- Dry, suffocative cough, especially in old people. Full of mucus but lacking strength to expectorate, worse every change of weather.

Dose: Baryta carbonica 30, 4 pills thrice daily for one month. Baryta is slow in action and bears repetition.

Chapter 13

Other Alternative Therapies

Many alternative therapies for high blood pressure focus on relaxation technique. Others are an attempt to get closer to the physiological roots of the problem, either by changing the person's habits or lifestyle, or by influencing the operation of the heart and blood vessels.

Different types of alternative therapies are:

- Acupressure
- Chinese herbalism
- Juice therapy
- Herbal therapy
- Body massage
- Yoga
- Aromatherapy
- Breathing and relaxation
- Mind and body medicine: Biofeedback, meditation, hypnosis
- Home remedies

ACUPRESSURE

An ancient system of massage aimed at encouraging *chi* (life energy) circulation throughout the body. It is regularly practiced by many Chinese people, particularly for self-treating common ailments and boosting the body's immune system.

Applying gentle pressure to several key points on the body may help improve circulation and reduce high blood pressure. The practitioner stimulates acupoints using her fingers, thumbs and even her feet and knee.

Pressure is applied directly down on to the skin or angles at the direction of the meridian's flow and acupoint on both sides of the body are massaged to balance *chi* flow. You should feel a slight discomfort when the acupoint is pressed.

Applying pressure on carefully chosen point of the body may help in relieving the symptoms associated with high blood pressure.

Following points are helpful in high blood pressure:

- **Pericardium 3:** Pressing pericardium 3 point may help relax the nervous system. Locate the point along biceps tendon at the elbow crease, in a direct line with your ring finger. Using thumb, apply firm pressure for one minute, then repeat on the other arm.

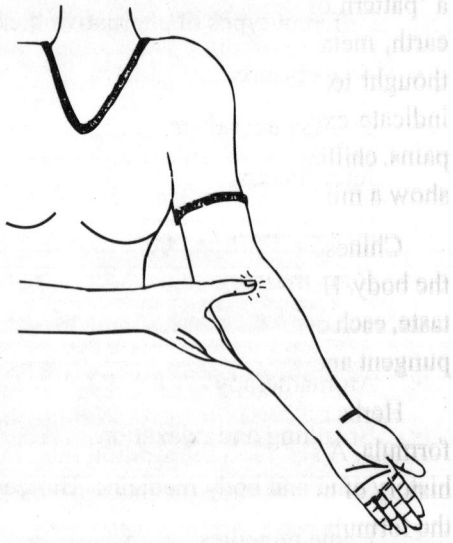

Fig. 29: Acupressure on Pericardium 3 point

- **Spleen 6 Point:** Pressure on spleen 6 point is four finger width up from the inner anklebone, near the edge of shinbone. Press gently with thumb for one minute, then repeat on the other leg.

In pregnancy this point is contraindicated.

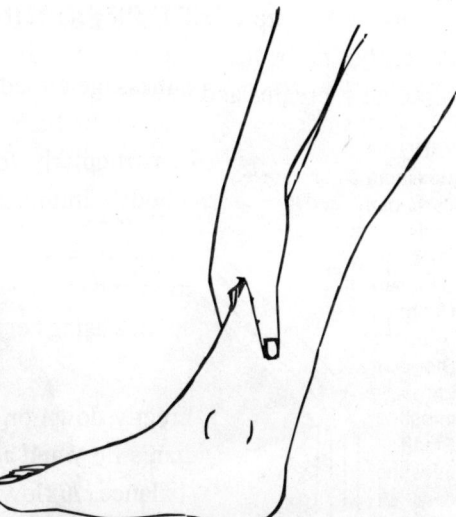

Fig. 30: Acupressure on Spleen 6 point

CHINESE HERBALISM

Traditional Chinese medicine regards the symptom as part of a 'pattern of disharmony' *YIN/YANG* and the five elements (fire, earth, metal, water and wood) theory are used. *Yang organs* are thought to "channel" energy – acute pain, sprains and headache indicate excess *Yang*. *Yin* organs 'hold' energy – dull aches and pains, chilliness and fatigue are signs of excessive *Yin*. Most people show a mixture of *Yin/Yang* symptoms.

Chinese herbal remedies are used to rebalance forces within the body. Herbs are classified under the five elements according to taste, each of which denotes a medicinal actions; sweet, sour, bitter, pungent and salty.

Herbs are rarely prescribed singly but are generally taken as a formula. A standard preparation may include 10–15 herbs with a history of treating a particular pattern of disharmony. Each herb in the formula has a different role, and each is classified according to its taste and temperature.

Remedies are usually taken as herbal teas, prepared in daily doses, but herbs may also be prescribe as pills, powders, pastes, ointments, creams and lotions.

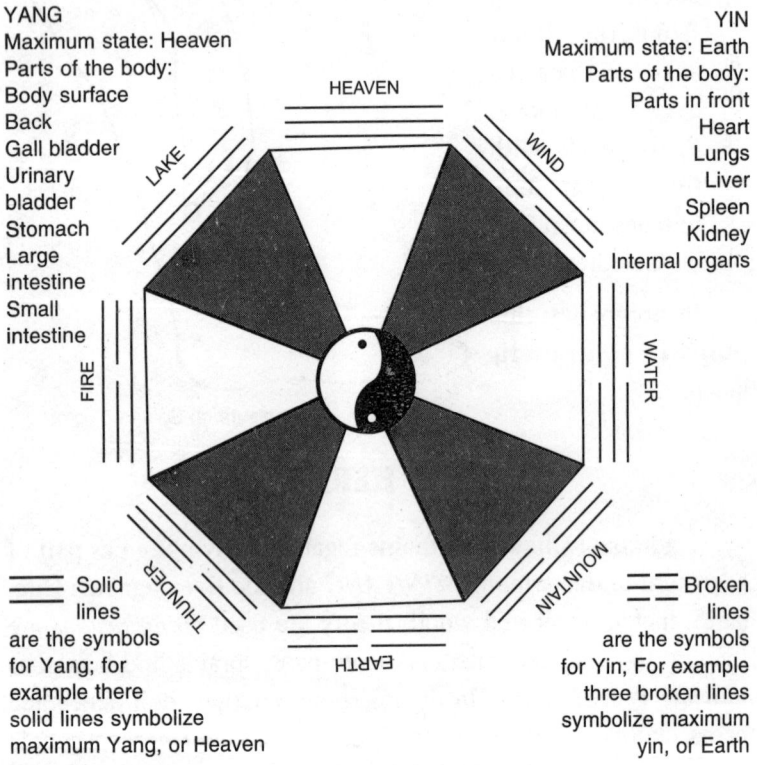

Fig. 31: Yin and Yang

Herbs for High Blood Pressure

Traditional Chinese healers treat high blood pressure by coupling acupuncture or acupressure with herbal therapy. Following herbs are useful for high blood pressure:

- Peony (Paeonia lactiflora)
- Eucommia bark (Eucommia ulmoides)
- Prunella (Prunella vulgaris)

- Tian Ma
- Rehmannia

Precautions

Always consult a practitioner who is fully qualified to prescribe herbal remedies. Seek medical advice before taking herbs in pregnancy, or if you have ever had hepatitis or other liver diseases.

JUICE THERAPY

The juice of fresh fruits and vegetables are the richest available food source of vitamins, minerals and enzymes. Usually, people just can't eat enough raw fruit and vegetables in a day to nourish the body. On most days, people probably can't find the time to eat enough fruits. But they certainly can find the time to drink their nutritional equivalent in a delicious, nutrient-rich glass of juice. That's why juicing is such an important addition to a busy lifestyle. Juice enable your body to easily assimilate the many valuable nutrients found in food. The quick and easy digestion of these foods, made possible by the enzymes, will give a greater energy and health.

Advantage of Juice Therapy

Juices make some of the very best dietary supplements available today. They are full of nutrients. These drinks are called as 'vitamin and mineral cocktails'. The body gets the nutrients needed for detoxification and the tissues in body absorb these nutrients. If one does not take these nutrients in his diet, he could become deficient in these.

The digestion of proteins and fats requires a lot of work. These processes can take many hours to complete. But it is estimated that fresh fruit and vegetable juices, which are already separated from fibre, can be assimilated in twenty to thirty minutes because they are easy to digest and absorb.

Juice is defined as a compound having water, flavors, pigments, enzymes, vitamins, minerals that promote healing, energy, and protection from disease. Juice should be a part of comprehensive approach of wellness. Juice therapy has worked to bring about recovery from illness for thousands of people.

Suggested Juice Recipes for High Blood Pressure

Potassium Broth—Mix

Handful spinach

Handful parsley

4–5 carrots + 2 stalks celery

Garlic Express—Mix

1 garlic clove

4–5 carrots

Handful parsley + 2 stalks celery

Sweet Magnesium Smoothie—Mix

1 ripe banana

1 pint blackberries

1 table spoon yeast

Drink this juice 1 hour before bedtime

Heaviest Soup—Mix

1 large tomato

2–3 garlic cloves

2 stalks celery

1 kale leaf

Calcium-Rich Cocktail—Mix

    4–5 carrots

    ½ apple

    Small handful parsley

Magnesium Drink—Mix

    4–5 carrots

    1 garlic clove

    Small handful parsley and 2 stalks celery

- Mix carrots, spinach, red beet, parsley and pumpkin
- Mix 300 ml of carrot juice and 200 ml of spinach juice to make 500 ml of the juice. This should be taken daily.

HERBAL THERAPY

Herbalism is a holistic medical system that seeks to restore the body's self-healing mechanism, or 'vital-force', and prescribes remedies tailored to the patient, not the system. Rather than treating symptoms in isolation, herbalism look for the cause of illness, such as poor diet, an unhealthy lifestyle or excessive stress, which may have overburdened the body's delicate balance.

Herbal remedies are extracted from flowers, leaves and other parts of a whole plant. Different parts of the same plant, for example the flowers and seeds, can have quiet different actions and if it is essential that the correct medicinal part of the plant is processed.

Disease attribute to a disruption in the maintenance of the body's state of harmony. Remedies promote healing by supporting the body's vital force in its effort to restore homeostasis.

Herbs are commonly dispensed as tinctures, made by steeping herbs in alcohol. Other remedies taken internally include tablets, infusions and decoctions, creams, lotions, oils, ointments are prescribed for external use.

Some common herbs for high blood pressure are:

Garlic (Allium Sativum)

Garlic lowers blood cholesterol and fat levels and reduces blood pressure. It is said to reduce spasms of the small arteries. It also slow down the pulse rate and modifies the heart rhythm. It has antibiotic and antiseptic action, and has ability to fight certain cancers.

Hawthorn berries (Crataegus)

It is used to treat many circulatory disorders, may help reduce high blood pressure. The herb may help in dilating coronary blood vessels, straightens heart's action and improves circulation. They also protect calcium levels and have a sedative effect on central nervous system. Hawthorn tea can be prepared at home by steeping the dried flowers and berries in hot water for 10 to 15 minutes.

Take hawthorn only under professional supervision.

Cactus Grandiflora

It is a cardiac herb with diuretic action as well. Hawthorn + Cactus + Garlic reduces blood pressure and blood cholesterol markedly within three months.

Lime Flowers

It is for nervous system as well as high blood pressure. It helps in dilation of constricted blood vessels and so reduces the pressure in the arteries.

Yarrow

This herb is of value in high diastolic pressure and all types of thrombosis. It dilates and tones arterioles and increases the peripheral blood pressure by 50%.

Mistletoe

It affects the capillaries and arterioles and reduces heart rate. It reduces blood pressure combined with other herbs.

Chamomile

It relaxes blood vessel walls. It also prevents the risk of thrombosis.

Valerian

It works with Chamomile and reduces blood pressure in stressed and anxious people.

Linden

It is of value in the type of high blood pressure causing a dull congestive headache because it has strong antispasmodic effect. This can be used as tea, thrice daily if appropriate.

Lavender

It is an antispasmodic herb with hypotensive properties. It is very useful in disorders like anxiety and stress. Use the essential oil of this herb, one drop on each temple twice daily.

Some other herbs like buckwheat, dandelion or parsley (used as diuretics) may also be given in high blood pressure.

Precautions

- Consult a qualified herbalist before taking any herb
- Consult a qualified herbalist before taking herbal medicine in cases of pregnancy, high blood pressure, heart disease and glaucoma
- Do not take Mille focium or medicinal doses of parsley during pregnancy
- Take hawthorn only under professional supervision

BODY MASSAGE

Massage may be the oldest and simplest from of Medical care. Ayurveda, the traditional Indian system of medicine, places great emphasis on the therapeutic benefits of massage with aromatic oils and spices.

Massage can aid relaxation, directly affecting the body systems that govern heart-rate, blood pressure, respiration and digestion. While it is not a cure for specific complaints the resulting sense of well-being from massage can lower the amount of circulating stress hormones, such as cortical and non-epinephrine, that can weaken the immune system.

All forms of touch are perceived through the skin, which is the body's largest sensory organ. Thousands of specialized receptors in the dermis (the second layer of skin) react to external stimuli, such as heat, cold and pressure, by sending messages through the nervous system to the brain. Gentle massage or stroking can release the endorphins which are body's natural pain killers and induce a feeling of comfort and well-being. Stronger, more vigorous massage may help to stretch, tense and uncomfortable muscles and ease stiff joints, improving mobility and flexibility.

Massage releases tension and reduces anxiety so that people feel more serene and better equipped to cope with the stress of life.

Regular sessions of massage can help lower blood pressure by promoting relaxation. Slow, stroking massage helps release muscles tension and may be effective, even in those who find it difficult to unwind, several studies proved that the massage can lower blood pressure temporarily, although it cannot control it permanently.

Procedure

Light vegetable oil or talcum power is usually used, so that hands glide over the skin. Essential oils may be added.

Other Alternative Therapies

Most therapists begin by massaging the back, followed by the neck and the back of the legs. However, there is no set order or procedure. The front of the legs, shoulders, arms and hands, neck and face are usually massaged next. Abdominal massage is not obligatory, but can be very pleasant if gently done.

Precautions

- Do not massage fractures, swellings, bruises, or skin infection, lumps and swelling should be checked by doctor

- Massage of the abdomen, legs and feet should not be given during the first three months of pregnancy

- Seek medical advice before having a massage if you have varicose veins, severe acute back pain, fever, thrombosis or phlebitis

YOGA

Yoga is a complete system of mental and physical training. It has been practiced for thousands of years in India as part of Ayurveda, and has now become popular

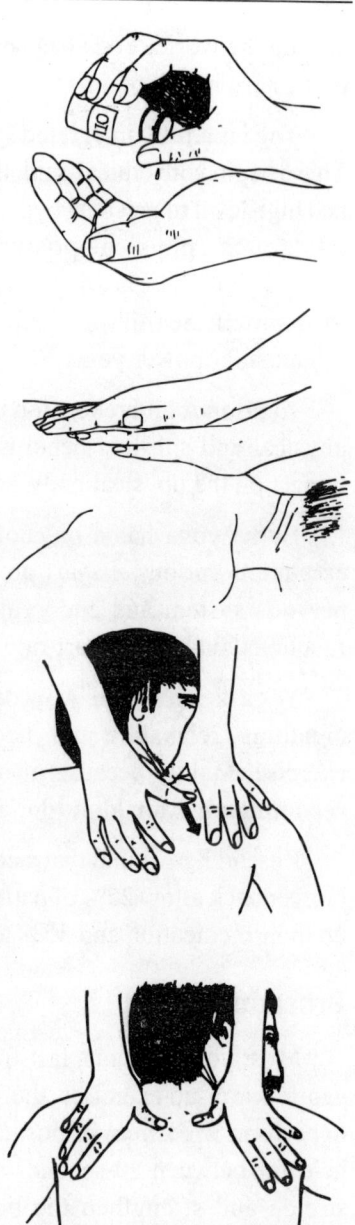

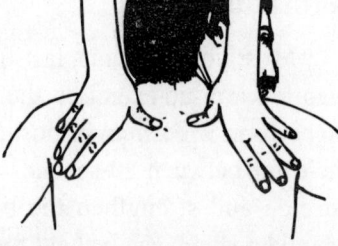

Fig. 32: Step by step procedure for body massage

around the world. Yoga has now been incorporated into a number of western health regimes.

Yoga is a fully integrated system controlling all aspects of life. These begin with ethical guidelines, including healthy eating habits and high level of personal hygiene and progress through the practice of *Asanas* (physical postures) and *Pranayama* (breathing techniques). There are many types of yoga, including yoga therapy to maintain health and help specific medical conditions and ashtanga, or power yoga.

Yogasanas and relaxation techniques were developed to bring physical and spiritual benefits. *Asanas* are designed to have an impact on the physical body, stimulating nerve centre and organs.

Hatha yoga has a physiological effect on muscle tone and escalation various *Asanas* are believed to affect the autonomic nervous system and endocrine glands, which regulate internal functions, including heart-rate and hormone production.

Yoga is powerful way of reducing stress, as it combines breathing, relaxation and meditation techniques and stretching exercise. Mainly because of its relaxing effects, **Yoga is highly recommended for high blood pressure**.

Researchers found that a combination of yoga, meditation and biofeedback allow 25% of patient with high blood pressure to give up their medication and 35% to reduce it.

Procedure

Most yoga sessions last from 1- 1½ hours. After undergoing gentle warm-up exercises, the yoga teacher shows the correct way to perform *yogasanas* or postures. Sitting and standing *asanas* are held for between 20 seconds and 2 minutes and are designed to stretch and strengthen the body. Inverted postures, such as a shoulder stand, can be held for longer. Counter-postures are often used in an *asana* to open the chest and free the neck may follow. A headstand are not advised in high blood pressure.

It is encouraged to be relaxed physically and mentally throughout the practice, to be conscious of while breathing and to remember, not to hold breath when practicing the *Asanas*. You should never be tempted to push yourself too far.

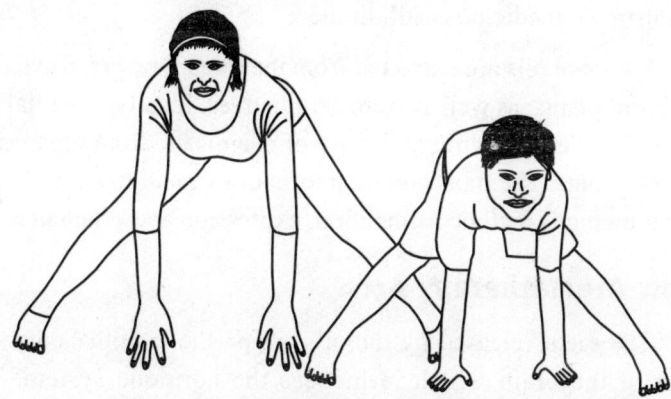

Fig. 33: Yogasanas for high blood pressure

Precautions

- Allow three hours after a meal before exercising
- Headstand and some other *asanas* are not advised if there are complaints of neck or back injury, high blood pressure, circulatory problem, heart disease or disorders of brain, ears or eyes
- Take care if you are practicing yoga during pregnancy or menstruation. Certain *Asanas* such as headstand should be avoided during pregnancy and during menstruation.

AROMATHERAPY

Herbal oils have been used since centuries in diverse cultures to treat illness and promote well-being and beauty. In ancient Egypt they were used. Aromatherapy over the centuries known to exist in

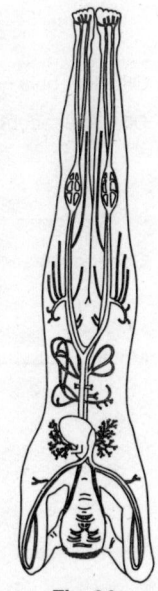

Fig. 34: A Yogasana

plants with the tradition of healing massage with oil. Modern aromatherapy practice is largely based on research by doctors in France, where essential oils are sometime prescribed as alternative to conventional medicine, though their use worldwide within mainstream medicine is still limited.

Essential oils are extracted from the roots, flowers, leaves and stalks of plants, as well as from certain trees. Ideally, essential oils should be derived without the use of chemicals, from organically grown plants. The most common form of extraction is distillation, other methods include maceration, expression and effeurage.

How Aromatherapy Acts

The scent released by the oils act on the hypothalamus, the part of the brain which influences the hormone system. The fragrance might be able to affect mood, metabolism, libido and stress levels.

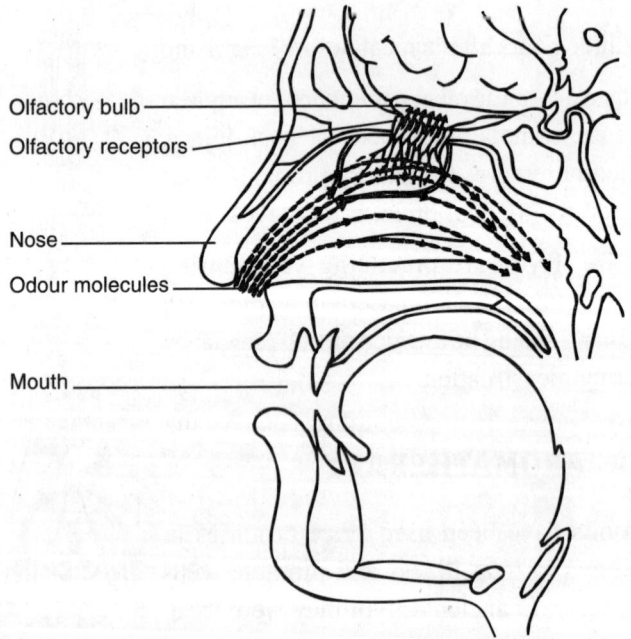

Fig. 35: The olfactory system

In theory, essential oils are absorbed into the body either through the pores of the skin during massage, or by inhalation through the nose. Molecules within the oils are said to enter through the bloodstream into the nervous system, influencing physical and emotional well-being.

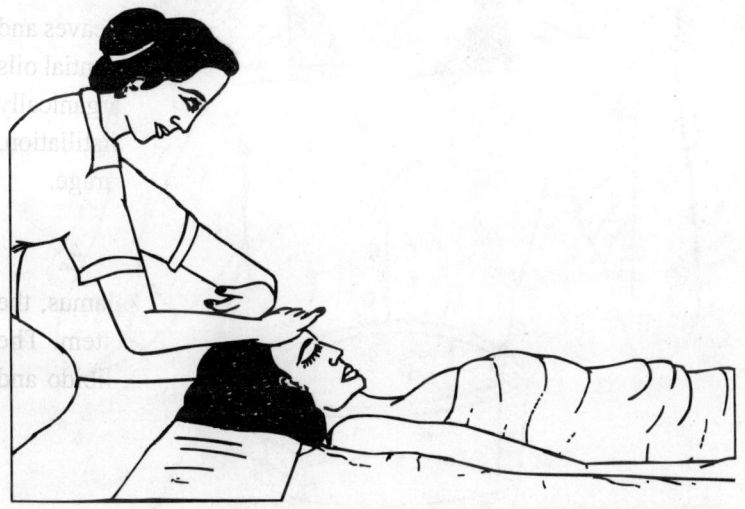

Fig. 36: Procedure of aromatherapy

A trained practitioner will use only high-quality oils, free from synthetic additives that may adversely affect the properties of an oil. The oils are diluted in a vegetable based carrier oil, such as almond or grape seed for massage, or blended in a lotion or cream for external application.

Aromatherapy massage is usually based on a Swedish massage technique, which aims to relieve tension in the body and improve circulation. Aromatherapy practitioners believe that oil molecules absorbed into the blood stream during massage pass efficiently through the body to the nervous system. The massage will also stimulate the lymphatic system, which helps to remove metabolic wastes from the body. In addition to massage, oils can be inhaled, vaporized or added to bath. Inhalations are recommended. Practitioners give specific oils or blends to use at home.

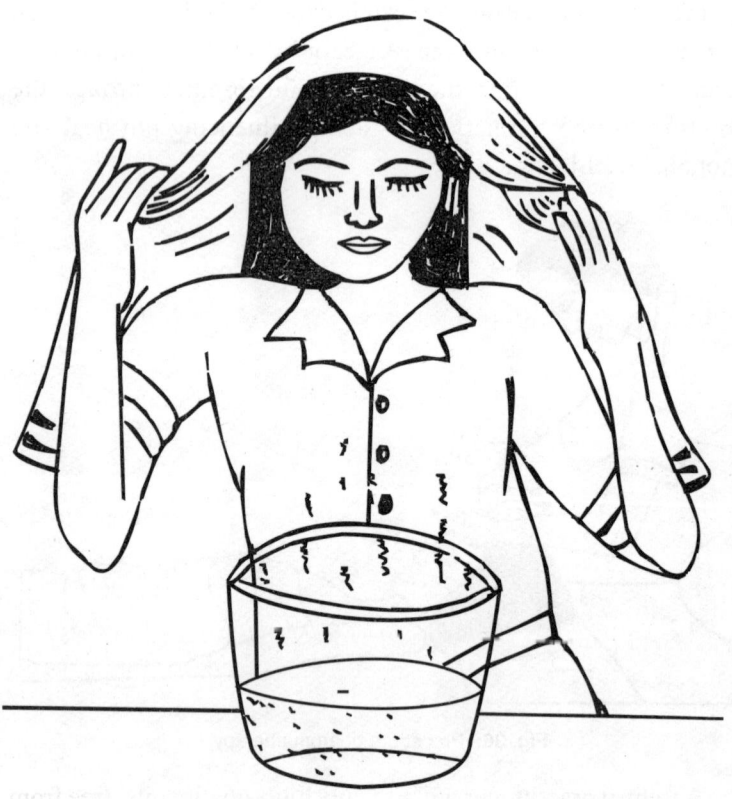

Fig. 37: Inhalation

For inhalation add 4 drops of essential oil to a bowl of steaming hot water and lean over the bowl with head covered by a towel and eyes closed. Inhale for up to 10 minutes. Alternatively, place 4–5 drops of oil on a tissue, hold it close to nose and take deep breaths. Do not inhale directly from the bottle. Inhalation are thought to be highly effective since olfactory receptors have direct links with the brain.

Essential oils for high blood pressure

Essential oil of **Lavender, Geranium, Sandalwood, Rose** or **Clary saga,** all are of good for high blood pressure because they have sedative qualities. Massage from these oil can help in complaint of high blood pressure.

Oils	Properties & Effects	Precautions
Lavender	**Main property** Sedative, Antidepressant, Antispasmodic, Antiseptic. It effect, nervous tension, helps in high blood pressure, palpitation, headache, digestive problems like diarrhea, colic, indigestion, flatulence, skin problems like acne, insect bites.	———
Sandalwood	**Main property** Sedative, Antiseptic Decongestant. Nervous tension – Helps in depression, sleeplessness, skin problems like acne, eczema. Respiratory problems – Sore throat, laryngitis, bronchitis.	———
Clary Sage	**Main property** Antispasmodic, painkiller sedative. Nervous tension – Helps in depression, anxiety, mental fatigue. Digestive problems – Indigestion and flatulence. Menstrual pain	Do not use during pregnancy. Avoid alcohol before and after use.

Precautions

- Make sure practitioner is qualified in case of pregnancy, epileptic convulsions or high blood pressure

- Use inhalations with care if there is tendency for asthma or prone to nosebleed
- Never use essential oils on the skin except lavender oil on burns and tea tree oil on insect bites
- Never swallow any oils, except under the supervision of a medically trained aromatherapist

BREATHING AND RELAXATION

Controlled breathing and the ability to relax at will are essential aspects of managing stress. Simple breathing exercises and muscle-relaxation technique mental effects mental stress, bringing therapeutic benefits such as lower heart-rate, reduce blood pressure and lower levels of stress hormone.

Breathing is involuntary and automatic, but since it can also be consciously controlled, it forms a bridge between mind and body. *'Pranayama'* in yoga is same thing because it helps in steady breathing and calm the body and mind. Abdominal breathing often practiced with muscle relaxation. These techniques calm both mind and body.

Theory of Breathing

With each breathing, oxygen is absorbed into the blood, enabling production of the energy that fuels body's function. Under stress, breathing tends to be rapid, using the top half of the lungs. This causes a drop in blood levels of carbon dioxide, which is needed to maintain blood acidity. This can lead to tiredness and anxiety and create tension in the upper back, shoulders and neck. Abdominal breathing, which allows full expansion of the lungs is a more effective and calm way to breath, and has the potential to benefit both physical and mental health.

RESPONSE TO STRESS

Adrenaline is released into bloodstream; heart rate and blood pressure increase

↓ Long term effect of Stress

High blood pressure; anxiety; insomnia; irritability

Relaxation & Breathing ↓

(Response to relaxation) Decreased adrenaline levels; lowers blood pressure; less stress on cardiovascular system

Table: Showing response of stress, and response of relaxation and breathing

What is Abdominal Breathing

In abdominal breathing the diaphragm is used. Diaphragm is a sheet of the chest cavity and the ceiling of the abdomen. On breathing in, the diaphragm contracts and moves downward. At the same time, the abdomen rises and the chest expands slightly as air is drawn in. On breathing out, the diaphragm relaxes and rises, making the space inside the chest cavity smaller and expelling air from the lungs.

Breathing Exercise

In the first exercise, the practitioners helps the person in mastering abdominal breathing. This is a gentle, relaxing technique, not necessarily 'deep' breathing. The technique customizes which allows the lungs to fill and empty with minimum effort. Once learnt, it can be practiced daily and should take around 10–15 minutes to complete. If overexertion is felt, stop and breath in normal way for a few minutes.

Procedure

• Tight clothing should be loosen. Sit in a comfortable position with a back support. Eyes should be closed if desired.

• Place one hand on the upper chest and the other on abdomen, just below breast bone. Notice which hand moves while breathing. If the hand placed on chest moves more than the one on abdomen, then breathing is mainly in the upper chest. Try

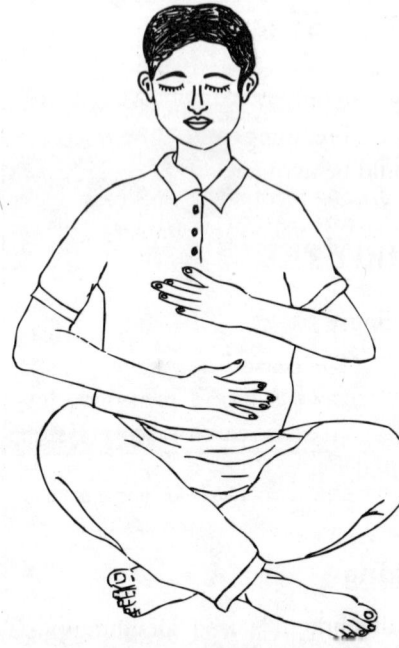

Fig. 38(a): Breathing exercise

to breath in a manner so that only lower hand moves.

• Both hands should be placed on abdomen below the ribs. Breathe in slowly through nose, allowing the abdomen to rise as the diaphragm moves down.

• Pause should be given for a few seconds between breaths, then breathe out slowly through nose, feeling the fall of abdomen as diaphragm relaxes. As

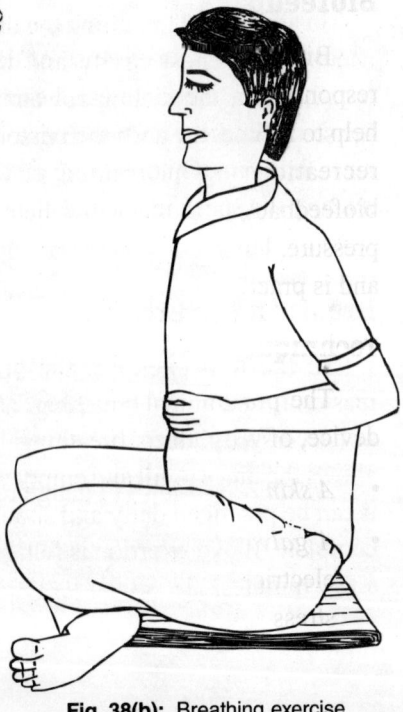

Fig. 38(b): Breathing exercise

much air as possible be expelled from should let out of your lungs.
- Repeat 3–4 times. Throughout the exercise, relaxation of muscles and concentration on breathing should be tried and any thought that comes should be avoided.

MIND AND SPIRIT THERAPIES

A number of method, including:
- Biofeedback
- Meditation
- Hypnotherapy: Call on the mind to relax the body and practicing over time with guidance from trained professionals, may help in lowering blood pressure.

Biofeedback

Biofeedback makes use of device that monitor physiological responses for example ear, heart and brain-wave patterns. It can help to recognize when the person is relaxed so that the feeling of recreation can be created at will. Studies have shown that biofeedback techniques may help people with mildly raised blood pressure. This technique is often used to treat stress-related ailments and is practiced in the UK, North America and Australia.

Technique

The practitioner will show you how to use the biofeedback device, of which there are several types:
- *A skin response* (ST) gauge registers heat changes in the skin
- *A galvanic skin response* (GSR) sensor, measures the skins electrical conductivity by the amount of sweat produced under stress

- *Electromyogrpahs* (EMGs) use auditory or visual signals to indicate muscle tension
- *Electroencephalographs* (ECGs) monitor heart rate

Once the sensors are in place, the signals that suggest relaxation are taught.

A state of relaxation is indicated by warm skin, low sweat-gland activity, high levels of *alpha* waves from the brain and a slow and even heart-rate.

Biofeedback practice takes at least six and a half-hours.

Precautions

Do not change the dosage of any medication during the course of biofeedback treatment without consulting a doctor.

MEDITATION

Techniques that quieten and focus the mind can help generate deep alpha brain-waves, which are associated with relaxation.

Meditation is intended to induce a state of profound relaxation, inner harmony and increased awareness. Various techniques can be used during meditation; all involve focusing the mind on a particular object or activity and disregarding distractions. Meditation has been shown to reverse the body's 'fight-or-flight' response to stress.

The state of meditation can be interpreted in various ways. It may be described as a condition in which the mind focuses on a thought or image; a non-judgemental receptiveness to whatever enters the mind; a state of 'relaxed awareness', or one in which the mind is empty. All this involves withdrawing from external reality and achieving deep relaxation and increased mental clarity.

In meditation, the brain-waves change to a distinctive alpha pattern linked with deep relaxation and mental alertness. Regular mediators can shift into the mode at will, which allows them to deal with stress efficiently and counter conditions such as high blood pressure and muscular pain.

Various schools of meditation favor particular techniques. This may be the rhythm of the breathing; or a mantra; or a physical object, such as a religious icon or a repetitive movement.

How to do it?

It is possible to self teach the technique of meditation from books, tapes or videos, but it would be probably easier to consult a teacher who will show, how to achieve a meditative state.

Whichever approach you choose, there are a few basic requirement for practicing meditation successfully:

- A quite environment where you can meditate without being disturbed
- A comfortable position, usually sitting which prevents one from becoming drowsy or falling asleep
- A focus for the mind to help it withdraw from external reality

The object of meditation is a state of 'passive awareness', in which mind is gently directed back to the focus of attention whenever it wanders, which it naturally does, slow breathing and an awareness of the breath entering and leaving the body also help to promote deep relaxation. It would be advisable to meditate on a daily basis for around 15–20 minutes, preferably at the same time of day. Morning is an ideal time.

Mantra meditation

A word or phrase is repeated continually, either silent or aloud. It may relate to individual's personal beliefs or it can simply be a positive statement.

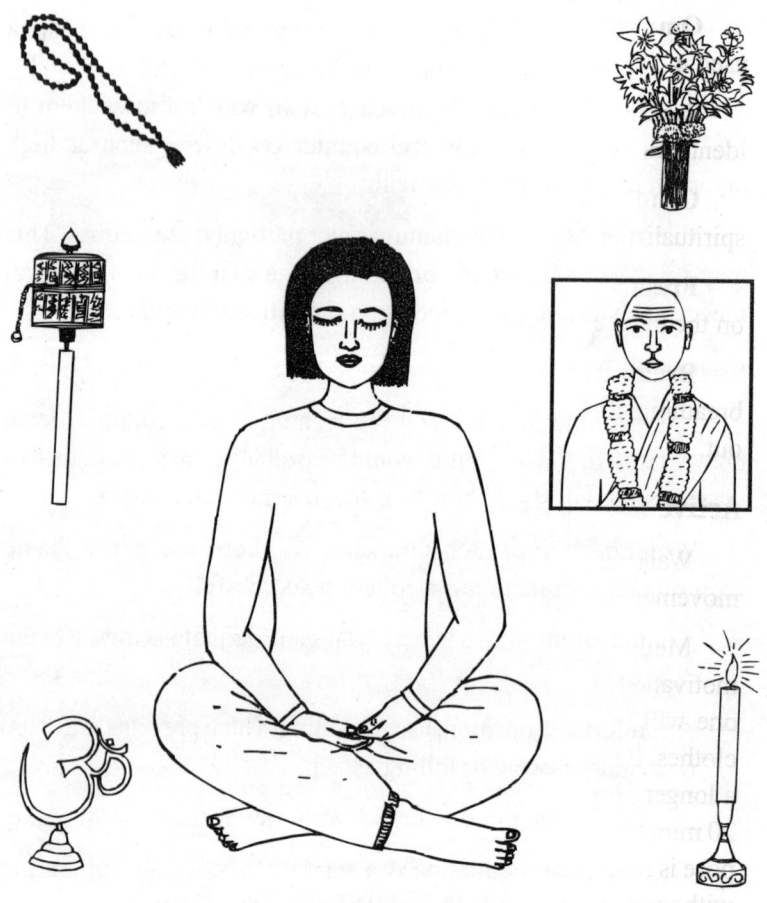

Fig. 39: Mantra meditation

Object meditation

An object conductive to meditation is chosen. The person concentrates on it, feeling its presence and focusing on its shape, weight, texture and other qualities.

Rosaries: Rosary beads may be used during meditation to count repetitions of a prayer.

Tibetan Prayer Wheel: Each rotation of the cylinder stands for one recitation of a mantra.

Om: For Hlindus, this is the most scared mantra. It is widely used in yogic meditation.

Portrait: An image of a spiritual leader, or someone individual identifies which may helps one to focus.

Candle: The flame is a symbol of the inner light of pure spirituality which is sought in meditation.

Fresh Flowers: These can have a calming and uplifting effect on the mind.

Breath awareness: The focus of attention should be on breathing. Count one or think of a peaceful word, with each breath out.

Active meditation

Walking, swimming and other activities involving rhythmic movement can focus the mind.

Meditation can be done with the help of discipline and motivation. First some quiet and warm place should be found where one will not be interrupted. While meditating wear comfortable clothes. Begin by sitting for a short time and gradually build up to a longer period. With practice, it should be possible to sit for 15–20 minutes at least once, and preferably twice a day. A cross-legged pose is not obligatory and you may prefer to sit on an upright chair, with your back straight. Eyes should be closed and relax. Breathing should be slow and rhythmical. Inhale through nose and feel the breath moving down to abdomen. Focus on the object of meditation. Allow the attention to be passive. When the mind wanders, simply acknowledge what is happening and then return to the focus of meditation. Try to stay as still as possible. In the end take a minute to become fully aware of the surroundings.

Precautions

Check with the doctor before starting meditation if there is any history of psychiatric problem.

HYPNOSIS

Technique of relaxing under hypnosis is done by trainer. The hypnotically induced state of relaxation may enable individual to re-enter the memory when it is necessary, helping one to cope more effectively with stressful situations or psychological conflicts. In hypnosis practitioners induce a state of consciousness akin to deep day dreaming, in which the patient is deeply relaxed and open to suggestions, and can be desensitized to fears, phobias or pain.

Principle of Hypnosis

Mind has different levels of consciousness. Under hypnosis, the conscious, rational part of the brain is temporarily bypassed, making the subconscious part, which influences mental and physical functions, extremely receptive to suggestion. During hypnosis, metabolism, breathing and heartbeat slow and the brain produces alpha waves.

Treatment with Hypnosis

The practitioner asks about individual's physical and mental health and his motivation to resolve any problem.

Individual lies on a reclining chair or couch and the practitioner talks in a slow soothing voice. Sometimes he might be asked to visualize something or to listen to a series of monotonous statements. The practitioner suggests that one feels heavy and relaxed, and that his eyes are closing.

Under hypnosis the practitioner may ask about past experiences to establish reasons for current problems. Alternatively, she may give suggestions to the patient's subconscious mind, aimed at over coming specific problems.

Precautions

- It is vital that you choose a trustworthy, qualified practitioner.
- Avoid hypnotherapy if you have severe depression, psychosis or epilepsy.

HOME REMEDIES

Adopt a healthy diet. Eat lots of fruit, vegetables and whole grains. Give up salty foods and add seasoning other than salt to meals. Drink less alcohol and caffeine. Quit smoking.

Exercise regularly to shed extra pounds and get blood flowing. Activities such as walking, jogging, cycling and swimming lower blood pressure over a long term.

Stress can't always be avoided but one can learn better ways to cope with it. Next time if stress is felt, ask innerself 'why' and then concentrate on solving the problem.

Garlic

Garlic is regarded as an effective means of lowering blood pressure. It reduces spasm of the small arteries. It also slows down the pulse rate and modifies the heart rhythm, besides relieving the symptoms of dizziness, numbness, shortness of breath and the formation of gas within the digestive tract.

It may be taken in the form of raw cloves or two to three capsules a day.

Indian Gooseberry (Amla)

Indian gooseberry (Amla) is another effective remedy for high blood pressure. A tablespoon each of fresh *Amla* juice and honey mixed together should be taken every morning in this condition.

Watermelon

A substance extracted from watermelon seed is said to have a definite action in dilating the blood vessels, which results in lowering the blood pressure. Watermelon is valuable safeguard against high blood pressure.

The seeds, dried and roasted, should be taken in liberal quantities.

Rauwolfia

Among the herbs, Rauwolfia is the best remedy for high blood pressure. Alkaloids of this drug, which have a direct effect on high blood pressure, have been isolated and are being widely used by practitioners of modern medicine. Practitioners of the Indian system of medicine have preferred to use the root of the drug in a powdered form.

Half a teaspoon of this drug, taken thrice a day, is very effective in high blood pressure.

Parsley

It contains elements which help maintain the elasticity of blood vessels, particularly, the capillaries. It keeps the arterial system in a healthy condition. Parsley is very useful in high blood pressure.

It may be taken as a beverage by immersing 20 gm of fresh parsley leaves gently in 250 ml of water for a few minutes. This may be drunk several times daily.

Lemon

Lemon is also regarded as a valuable food to control high blood pressure. It is a rich source of Vitamin C which is found both in the juice and peel of the fruit. This vitamin is essential for preventing capillary fragility.

Potato

Potatoes, specially boiled potatoes are a valuable food for lowering blood pressure. When boiled with their skin, they absorb very little salt. Potatoes are rich in potassium but not in sodium salts. The magnesium present in the vegetable exercises beneficial effect in lowering blood pressure. Thus they can form a useful addition to a salt-free diet, recommended for patients with high blood pressure.

Grape Fruit

It is useful in preventing high blood pressure. The Vitamin C content in the fruit is helpful in toning up the arteries.

Rice

Rice has a low-cholesterol, low-fat and low-salt content. It makes a perfect diet for high blood pressure person. Calcium, present in brown rice, soothes and relaxes the nervous system and helps in relieving the symptoms of high blood pressure.

Vegetable Juices

Raw vegetable juices, taken separately or in combination, are also beneficial in the treatment of high blood pressure.
(Please see juice therapy section for more details).

Chapter 14

Special Considerations

Some medical conditions, require special consideration with regard to high blood pressure. Those who require special attention include people suffering from particular illness or taking certain kinds of drugs, children, pregnant women and elderly.

PREGNANCY

High blood pressure occurs in about 1% of all pregnant women and can cause harm to both, the baby and mother. However, with early diagnosis and treatment, harm can be prevented. That's why nurses and doctor keep measuring blood pressure all through pregnancy.

Blood pressure normally falls during pregnancy due to a generalized relaxation of the mother's blood vessels. It reaches a low point about half-way (from 14 to 27 weeks) through the pregnancy and then slowly rises until baby is born (which is normally at 38 to 42 weeks) and then slowly rises to regain its usual level before pregnancy.

During pregnancy, not only the woman needs oxygen but her developing baby also requires equal amounts of it. The body therefore makes more blood to carry enough oxygen for both. Therefore, the total volume of blood rises rapidly during the first 12 to 13 weeks of pregnancy. A rise in blood volume should cause a rise in blood pressure. To prevent this, placenta (which links mother's blood supply with baby's) releases hormones mainly progesterone which relaxes the walls of the veins and small arteries which become larger to make room for this increased blood volume, without any rise in the blood pressure. Because of this heart doesn't have to pump so hard and the blood pressure falls. Because of fall in blood pressure he/she may feel dizzy or faint when they get up out of a chair or from lying down.

A blood pressure of 140/90 mmHg or more is conventionally considered to be high blood pressure in pregnancy. Some women actually found out that the blood pressure is high during pregnancy, but this is because it has been that way for some time and they have not had it checked before. In this situation it is purely coincidental and not really related to pregnancy; it just happens to be detected while in pregnancy.

High blood pressure developing for the first time during pregnancy develops over a very short time, never more than a few weeks and occasionally over a few hours. During this time it can cause very serious damage to small arteries, particularly in the kidneys and brain. The same kind of damage may occur in other people suffering from high blood pressure, but only at much higher levels of blood pressure, and usually over much longer period.

Conditions that cause High Blood Pressure During Pregnancy

Three conditions may produce high blood pressure during pregnancy. The management of high blood pressure during pregnancy is the same as for anyone else who is diagnosed with high blood pressure, although the choice of drugs may be different in allopathic treatment.

Special Considerations

1. Chronic High Blood Pressure

Chronic high blood pressure means high blood pressure starting before pregnancy. Almost all women of childbearing age with this condition have, *"essential high blood pressure"* that is high blood pressure without a cause that can be identified. Women are hypertensive before they become pregnant can remain hypertensive during their pregnancy. Sometimes in the last few months of the pregnancy. This poses a danger to mother and fetus alike.

2. Gestational High Blood Pressure

It is defined as high blood pressure without swelling or protein loss in the urine, occurring in a mother who had normal blood pressure before conception. About 25 percent of women expecting their first baby develop slightly raised blood pressure in the last three months of pregnancy. There is no damage to kidney and no protein appearing in the urine on testing. It usually arises in the late stage of pregnancy and restores within 2 weeks after delivery. It often recurs in later pregnancies. This condition is also known as pregnancy-induced hypertension (PIH) or pregnancy-related hypertension.

3. Pre-eclampsia and Eclampsia

The Pre-eclampsia arises only during pregnancy and disappears after the foetus is delivered. Pre-eclampsia is defined as the appearance of high blood pressure, ankle swelling and protein in the urine during the second half of pregnancy. Pre-eclampsia occurs most often in the first pregnancy and uncommonly in subsequent pregnancies. It affects about five percent of women in their first pregnancy and is defined as a blood pressure of over 160/90 mmHg protein in urine.

Eclampsia literally means 'flashing lights'. In practice it means fits (seizures) caused by brain damage which is in turn caused by very high blood pressure that develops very fast, usually in pregnancy. Sufferer of eclampsia suddenly looses consciousness, the whole body shakes uncontrollably, with clenched teeth and severe spasm of all muscles only for a minute or two but seems much longer. Eclampsia is very dangerous both to the mother and to the unborn child.

Eclampsia is preceded by pre-eclampsia, either by several weeks of slowly rising blood pressure or by dramatic warning signs like pain in the upper abdomen caused by congestion of the liver, severe persistent headache and blurred vision.

There is often a decrease in the output of urine or a increase in the blood of dietary waste products normally eliminated by the kidneys. In addition, the growth of the fetus in the womb may be retained. If left untreated, pre-eclampsia can progress into a very serious condition of *lampsia eclampsia*. Pre-eclampsia may cause pre-mature birth.

About two-third of women with severe pre-eclampsia and nearly three-quarters of those with mild pre-eclampsia have no problems with raised blood pressure in their second pregnancy.

Cause

The exact cause of this condition is not yet fully understood, but it likely originates in the placenta as a result of a decreased blood flow to the womb (uterus). The placenta has its own arteries. In pre-eclampsia these arteries do not penetrate well in the walls of the uterus (womb) and they seem to be narrowed by plaques of cholesterol and blood clots in much the same way as the coronary and leg arteries are in 'ordinary' high blood pressure. This reduces placental blood supply, which induces raised blood pressure throughout the body, and reduces blood flow to liver and kidneys.

Pre-eclampsia occurs most often in the first pregnancy and uncommon in subsequent pregnancies. There is an inherited tendency for pre-eclampsia, it tends to run in families, that is why doctors ask about blood pressure in near relatives, particularly in the mother or sisters. Researchers found that out of 248 women whose mother had suffered an eclamaptic fit, 1 in 4 had pre-eclampsia in their first pregnancy and 1 in 50 of these women had an eclamptic fit, so their risk was increased to 20 fold.

Pre-eclampsia occurs more often in mothers who already have raised blood pressure (means chronic high blood pressure) chronic kidney disease and diabetes before they conceive. The chances of its occurrence increases in mothers at the extremes of childbearing age, that is women over 40 years or teenagers.

Diagnosis

Regular blood pressure check up are especially important during pregnancy.

Urine test for protein—Urine normally contains only water with a large variety of rather simple waste products, mainly urea and salt, dissolve in it. Proteins are normally filtered out and retained by your kidneys and so do not appear in urine when blood pressure rises in pre-eclampsia. It rises much faster than high blood pressure in people who are not pregnant. Kidneys have had less time to adapt to the new higher level of blood pressure and so are more easily damaged and therefore damaged kidneys begin to leak protein in urine. The amount of protein in urine is roughly proportional to the serverity of the damage done to kidneys.

Sometimes patient may be asked to collect all the urine which is passed in 24 hours, to measure the total protein lost in urine throughout the day. This should be less than 300 mg in 24 hours. Some people loose protein in urine from time to time without any damage to kidney.

In severe pre-eclampsia, the level of protein in blood falls due to protein loss in urine. The blood cannot then retain all the water it contains; some leaks through the walls of the capillaries to the other parts of the body, making them swell which is known as edema. This swelling first becomes obvious in legs.

Management and treatment

Management of blood pressure during pregnancy depends on time and duration of pregnancy and type of high blood pressure.

Generally, the blood pressure rises for the first time after 36 weeks of pregnancy and it is usually best to deliver the baby and therefore labor is induced early. If blood pressure starts rising between 24 and 28 weeks, doctors often try to control it with or without blood pressure lowering drugs so that the baby is more mature when born and has a better chance of survival. Doctors vary in their opinions on how high blood pressure should be before the starting treatment.

Stress can affect blood pressure in some people and pregnant women usually need more rest than before. So proper modification in their work life is to be made.

Patients with chronic high blood pressure during pregnancy are often managed by asking them to increase the amount of rest they are getting at home. Drugs that lower elevated pressure are then added as necessary. Delivery is undertaken if the blood pressure is still not controlled or the foetus shows evidence of distress or electively, when the foetus is mature. Treatment of chronic high blood pressure does not prevent the added development of pre-eclampsia and doctor should be constantly watchful in this regard.

Women with gestational high blood pressure are managed in the same manner as those with chronic high blood pressure. Patient with gestational high blood pressure have a higher than average chance of developing high blood pressure later in life.

Women with mild pre-eclampsia can be managed with bed rest and drugs that lower elevated pressures. Women with severe pre-eclampsia require treatment of their elevated blood pressure and urgent delivery of the baby as they will not improve until the pregnancy is ended. After delivery most symptoms of pre-eclampsia may disappear rapidly. Pre-eclampsia stops after the birth of bably, although occasionally they may persist up to 6 months.

Allopathic Drugs for High Blood Pressure During Pregnancy

In pregnancy, there is a severe limit to the choice of blood pressure-lowering drugs. Most doctors begin medication that lowers elevated pressure when the mother's diastolic blood pressure is 100 mmHg or greater. The goal is usually a diastolic pressure of 80 to 90 mmHg because lower blood pressure may be dangerous for the foetus.

The *methyldopa*, *hydralzine* and *beta-blockers* (*oxprenolol, atenolol* and *labetolol*) are the blood pressure-lowering drugs, that have been well studied for use in pregnancy and are considered to be effective without endangering the development of the foetus. The blood pressure lowering drugs are most likely to use either methyldopa or beta-blockers.

Methyldopa is an old drug which, although have some side-effects, have a good track record for safety and effectiveness at all stages of pregnancy. Beta-blockers are well tolerated and apparently without risk to the baby after 24 weeks, before 24 weeks they may slow down the baby's growth and so should be avoided. Atenolol is probably best avoided because it may result in underweight babies. If these drugs are ineffective then most doctor would admit women with pre-eclampsia to hospital for treatment with hydralazine (a vasodilator drug).

Allopathic therapy usually begins with single drug – and then second and third drugs are added if necessary. If blood pressure cannot be controlled with these drugs then delivery should be undertaken for the mother's safety.

Avoid

Two types of drugs – Diuretics and Angiotensin Converting Enzyme (ACE) inhibitors, are **usually avoided** during pregnancy. Diuretics may increase the risk of low birth weight infants. ACE inhibitors such as *captopril* and *enalapril*, may cause growth retardation. Other agents, including *minoxidil* and *calcium antagonists* (diltiazem and verapmil) are not yet considered suitable for use in pregnancy because their safety during pregnancy has not been proved yet.

During Breast Feeding

Blood pressure-lowering drugs are taken after delivery by mothers whose breast contain milk is in small amounts. However, infants are routinely and successfully breast fed from mother taking *methyldopa hydralazine,* and *beta-blockers.* Diuretics are still avoided for treatment of high blood pressure after delivery as these drugs may decrease the amount of milk produced by the mother.

ORAL CONTRACEPTIVE

Oral contraceptive are the most popular form of temporary birth control measures. Oral contraceptive must be used with caution, however, because they sometimes cause adverse effects, including high blood pressure.

There are some medical situations in which oral contraceptives would usually not be prescribed, these are:

- Women over 35 year, who smoke and have a high risk of cardiovascular disease
- Oral contraceptives should not be prescribed to women with a history of stroke, heart attack, liver disease, known or unknown, suspected breast cancer, any estrogen-dependent tumour and abnormal uterine bleeding

- It should not be given during pregnancy or expected pregnancy
- It should not be given with a medical history of thrombophlebitis—the formation of blood clots in the veins.

Blood pressure rises a little in virtually all women who take estrogen-containing oral contraceptives. This rise usually starts 3 to 9 months after beginning the pill. Unfortunately, in about 5% of women over a 5-years of pill use, the rise is enough to push the blood pressure beyond the 140/90 mmHg level. In some women pills will cause severe high blood pressure. The exact cause by which oral contraceptives increases blood pressure is still unknown. Most women gain weight when put on the pill. For this, salt and water retention in body tissue has been suggested as the cause of their increased blood pressure. The incidence of high blood pressure is lower when "mini-pills" containing lower doses of estrogen are used.

High blood pressure is not an absolute reason to avoid used oral contraceptive, but other methods of contraception are preferable if individual has high blood pressure. If some one is unable to use another method, then medication may be prescribed for high blood pressure in addition to the oral contraceptive to lower the blood pressure.

Precaution with Contraceptive Pills

In normal circumstances the following precautions should be taken for the safe use of oral contraceptive:

- The lowest effective dose of estrogen (mini-pills) should be used
- These pills should not be taken for more than 6 month at a time
- The blood pressure should be checked regularly in every 2 months

- The blood pressure should be measured whenever the women feels ill
- If blood pressure rises, the pills should be stopped if possible and another form of contraceptive should be used
- If blood pressure does not return to normal within 6 months of stopping the pill, additional investigation and treatment are needed
- Studies show that the usually prescribed dose of postmenopausal estrogens, alone or in combination with progesterone have no effect on blood pressure

ELDERLY PEOPLE

As one gets old his your blood pressure rises and the risk of heart attack and strokes becomes correspondingly greater. High blood pressure is considered to be a major risk factor for the development of heart and vascular diseases in older people. Older people do have a higher frequency of other conditions, including diabetes and arthritis.

56% of men and 52% of women over the age of 65 years have a blood pressure higher than it should be. The systolic pressure increases with age. Although it was thought that the diastolic pressure was more important, in older people, the systolic pressure indicates the level of risk slightly better. Thus, the systolic pressure is now given more importance in deciding when to start treatment.

In some cases, the systolic pressure can increase without any change in the diastolic pressure. For example, 170/80 mmHg, this type of high blood pressure is called **isolated systolic hypertension**.

High blood pressure itself causes no complaints or symptoms in its early stage. However, if the high blood pressure is severe or remains untreated for a long time, it may cause damage to the heart, kidney or brain. For example, damage to the heart may cause shortness of breath, swelling of the feet, getting up more frequently during the night to pass urine and sometimes pain in the chest. There are a number of factors that can lead to cardiac disease, stroke or an aneurysm.

In older people, high blood pressure is the most treatable risk factor for heart or vascular disease. The risk associated with an increased blood pressure is in fact greater in the elderly patient than the younger patient.

Causes

Most elderly person (90–95%) with high blood pressure have "essential" high blood pressure. In elderly, some additional factors come into play. 5% to 10% elderly with high blood pressure have a "secondary" form of high blood pressure that is caused by dysfunction of the kidneys or the adrenal glands or of the blood vessels.

Over age the major blood vessels become less elastic and more rigid. This increased rigidity leads to an increase in the systolic blood pressure and play the major role in the prevalence of high blood pressure in old age group.

When the diagnosis is made, a detailed physical examination should be made by doctor to determine the condition of heart and blood vessels. Laboratory test will include urine and blood sample, to evaluate the function of kidneys and the blood sugar levels, as well as possibly a chest x-ray and an electrocardiogram.

Management

It has been proved that 65 to 85 years old with high blood pressure who have taken medication for their blood pressure suffer fewer strokes and are less likely to have heart failure than those who do not receive medication.

Patient with milder high blood pressure that is systolic pressure between 140 and 160 mmHg, may only require observation and general health management without treatment unless the physical examination or blood tests reveal damage to the heart, brain, kidneys or blood vessels. The treatment part on persons with medical history and symptoms along with physical examination and laboratory test results.

Treatment for high blood pressure is the same, whatever the age. A old person with high blood pressure initially advice to follow lifestyle changes. Obese patients are adviced to loose weight. Because there is difficulty in loosing weight for older individuals, they are advised to follow a balanced diet instead and to maintain their present weight. Alcohol should be restricted if blood pressure is high. Salt should be reduced in the diet. Smoking should be stopped as it causes further damage to heart and blood vessels. Exercise is generally healthy. As much as possible walking or other form of aerobic exercise is generally healthy. As much as possible walking or other form of aerobic exercise should be used to stay in shape and may be helpful to control blood pressure.

Allopathic Drugs

Treatment for high blood pressure is the same, whatever age may be. A diuretic is usually preferred to start treatment for high blood pressure in the elderly. There is a trend for the thiazide diuretics and the calcium channel blockers to be more effective while the ACE inhibitors and the beta-blockers are less effective, in older patients. Sometimes, two different drugs in low dose may be needed rather than any one drug in high dose. In order to limit side-effects, the lowest possible dose will be prescribed. Medication should not be stopped without advise of the physician because this might result in a sudden and a dangerous rise in blood pressure.

CHILDREN

Severely raised blood pressure in children is rare. It is associated with significant kidney conditions. Overweight children and those children with a strong family history of high blood pressure may have slightly raised blood pressure. Very rarely, children of high blood pressure can be the result of autosomal dominant polycystic kidney disease. If parents have high blood pressure, then their children are at risk of developing this condition too. In this condition make sure that the child's diet is low in salt and do not let them eat too many chips or other salted snacks. It is also imperative not to let them go fat.

HIGH BLOOD PRESSURE WITH DIABETES

Diabetes is a disease in which the quality of sugar (glucose) in the blood is elevated. Blood glucose level is maintained by the action of several hormones but mainly by insulin which is secreted by pancreas. Two types of diabetes are there:

1. **Type 1 diabetes—Insulin dependent diabetes mellitus (IDDM):** Pancreas don't produce enough insulin, the blood sugar goes up. It starts at young age usually in people below 20 years of age.
2. **Type 2 diabetes—Non insulin dependent diabetes mellitus (NIDDM):** The body produces insulin but the insulin doesn't work properly, the blood sugar rises. It usually starts later in life, after 40 years of age. People with this problem still produce insulin but for various reasons their insulin is not able to decrease blood sugar. Moreover, the quantity of insulin produced also diminishes with age.

Food is broken down in the gut and transformed into glucose (sugar), the main source of energy for all cells throughout the body and the only source of energy for brain cells. In diabetes, the chemical pathways for both; production and use of glucose fail to work properly.

People with high blood pressure are perhaps more likely to develop diabetes than other people and high blood pressure is more common in people who have diabetes than in the rest of the population. If both the conditions co-exsist, there is increased risk of developing damage to the eyes and kidneys, coronary heart disease and stroke. This is true if the blood pressure is only moderately raised. Rigorous control of high blood pressure is however very important for people with diabetes.

About 50% of diabetics have high blood pressure too and about 15% of high blood pressure patients have problem elevated blood sugar. The combination of high blood pressure and diabetes increase the chances of developing the complications. Further more, once complications are present, high blood pressure in diabetes increase the severity.

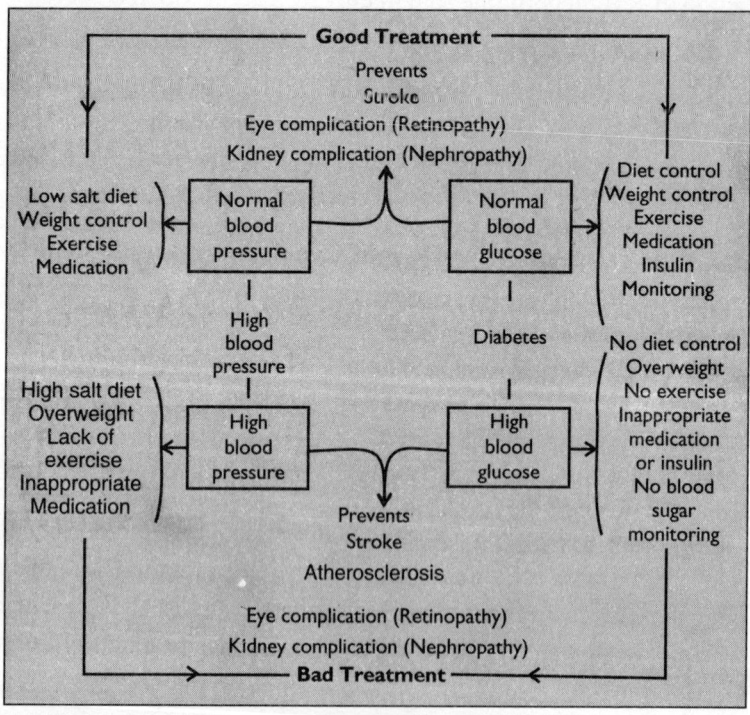

Table showing high blood pressure with diabetes

Diabetes affects blood vessels at two levels—large arteries and small vessels like arterioles and capillaries. Diseased large arteries progressively obstruct blood flow to the heart, brain and legs. They can cause angina, heart attack, strokes and cramps in legs (claudication) during exercise. Obstruction of small vessels mainly affects the eyes and kidneys. The retina, at the back of the eye, is most affected by diabetes. Obstruction of small vessels in the kidney eventually cause kidney failure.

Two types of high blood pressure can be associated with diabetes—essential high blood pressure and high blood pressure associated with renal disease. Essential high blood pressure in diabetics is probably of the same origin as in non-diabetics. In high blood pressure associated with renal disease, the kidney doesn't function normally and proteins are leaked from blood into the urine. Thus, renal disease in diabetics leads to high blood pressure and high blood pressure can worsen the renal problem. This is a vicious circle with serious consequences.

Management

There are many advantages in controlling high blood pressure strictly, in diabetics. Good control of high blood pressure decreases protein loss in urine and slows the rate of kidney function deterioration and the vicious circle can be broken. Good control of high blood pressure in diabetes also decreases the risk of stroke and the progression of retinopathy.

Apart from maintaining good glucose control efforts should be made to control weight, cholesterol levels needs to be checked and treated if raised. Decreased salt intake has added benefit because salt retention is a specific problem in diabetes.

Many doctors believe that all diabetics with diastolic pressure at or above 90 mmHg should be treated for high blood pressure even if there are no vascular complications.

Allopathic Treatment

Certain drugs should be avoided:

- Non-steroidal anti-inflammatory agents such as ibuprofen, naproxen or indomethacin can have an adverse effect on kidney function in diabetes
- Corticosteroids such as cortisone, prednisone increase the control over blood sugar
- Oral decongestants in cold remedies have effects similar to noradrenaline, to which diabetics are particularly sensitive

All these drugs can increase both blood pressure and blood sugar.

Several drugs can be used to treat high blood pressure in diabetics. There is evidence that one class of drugs—the ACE inhibitors, is better than other drugs in preventing kidney and eye damage. Several studies have shown that these ACE inhibitors decreases albumin leakage in the urine of diabetics. ACE inhibitors can increase blood potassium and sometimes make the potassium too high (hyperkalemia). For the most people with diabetes **ACE inhibitors are probably the first choice.**

Thiazide diuretics tends to reduce even further the body's ability to deal with glucose. Thiazide diuretics can increase blood sugar level when administered in high doses. They can elevate cholesterol and triglycerides too, when administered in high doses. However, thiazide diuretics particularly in low doses, are still an acceptable choice for treating high blood pressure in diabetics and are frequently useful in association with ACE inhibitors.

Beta-blockers can cause problems in diabetics. In some people beta-blocker drugs suppress the warning symptoms produced by hypoglycemia (low blood sugar level). The usual warning signs of hypoglycemia are dizziness, sweating, mental confusion etc. Hypoglycemia can lead to unconsciousness. So this could obviously be dangerous. Beta-blockers should be avoided if there is any suspicion about low blood sugar level.

Calcium antagonist, when first taken may increase blood sugar slightly when first taken, they don't do so with long-term use. They are also an excellent choice in the treatment of high blood pressure with diabetes.

Alpha-blockers don't affect blood sugar and they have advantageous effects on lipid, so they are good choice for most diabetics. The tendency of some diabetics suffer with blood pressure may worsen and pressure may become too low on standing from sitting position known as orthostatic hypotension.

Vasodilators have no bad effects on blood sugar. They increase the heart rate and cause fluid to be retained in the body when used alone. They are usually given with beta-blockers and diuretics.

Table: Medication for High Blood Pressure with Diabetes

First-line medication: In order of preference ACE inhibitors or calcium antagonists or alpha-blockers.

Second-line medications: Thiazide-like diuretics or beta-blockers (used with precautions).

Fall-back medications: Centrally acting drugs and vasodilators (when other drugs are contraindicated).

HIGH BLOOD PRESSURE WITH ASTHMA AND OTHER CHEST DISEASE

Asthma narrows airways and causes difficulty in breathing. Doctor will suspect asthma in anyone who has recurrent episodes of coughing, wheezing, shortness of breath or chest tightness. Other causes are a history of allergies and asthma affecting members of the family. There are two ways in which asthma present's itself in 2 stages: The first is inflammation of the linings of airways, so that they become swollen and produce too much mucus. The second, inflammation further makes airways very twitchy and irritable, which means that the spiral muscles that surrounds them tighten up (spasm) and narrow them still further when person come across anything that starts their coughing.

Anyone with above symptom should have their lung function checked to see if they have asthma. This usually involves taking a series of peak flow measurements over a week or so. Taking these measurements is very simple all you have to do is to blow as hard and as fast as possible into a small device called a **peak flow** meter and the result can then be read on its scale. The result can then be compared with the expected value for age, sex and height—if the reading is 25% or more below the expected value, then the trouble may be there and perhaps more readings are necessary to see asthma is there.

In allopathy inhalers are used during a attack of asthma. There are many different type of inhalers, best known as salbutamol, and terbataline. They work by relaxing the spiral muscles, which in turn allows the tightened airways to open up. They generally have a very rapid and easily recognized effect, so people are often tempted to overuse them. They have little or no effect on blood pressure.

However, if they are taken too much they can cause disturbances of heart rhythm which can be serious particularly in people who already have high blood pressure.

The most important point is that you cannot take beta-blockers if you have any form of wheeze, asthma or similar breathing difficulties with high blood pressure, but there is no problem in regards other allopathic antihypertensive drugs. Because a serious side-effect of beta-blockers is narrowed lung airways in people with asthma. Any use of beta-blockers can be very dangerous for any of these people, even a single dose can cause very severe tightening of the airways. ACE inhibitor (allopathic drug high blood pressure) can cause a dry, irritating cough, but this is not usually associated with breathlessness. The cough will disappear once you stop taking the tablets and there are plenty of alternative treatments.

HIGH BLOOD CHOLESTEROL LEVEL

Cholesterol is an essential component of all body cells and of many important circulating chemicals in the blood. It is present in large quantities in some foods such as egg yolk, kidneys, liver, other meat and fish oils. But cholesterol is formed in the body from the many different sorts of fats and oil that is available in your diet. If there is a surplus, most of this is stored in the liver, but some remains circulating in the blood.

The concentration of cholesterol in the body matters because the higher it is, the more of it is deposited as waxy plaques on the wall, of arteries—the coronary arteries (supplying blood to the heart), the aorta, the arteries of brain and leg arteries. The plaque, causes the arteries to narrow, which means blood clots are more likely to form and this can lead to partial or complete destruction of the organs supplied by these arteries.

Blood cholesterol, normally means total cholesterol. Of three different cholesterol-containing substances.

- High Density Lipoprotein (HDL)
- Low Density Lipoprotein (LDL)
- Very Low Density Lipoprotein (VDL)

HDL cholesterol is 'good' cholesterol because HDL is the form in which cholesterol is transported in the blood before storage in the lever, LDL and VLDL cholesterol are 'bad' cholesterol, the source of waxy plaques on the walls of the aorta, coronary arteries, brain arteries and leg arteries. LDL and VLDL are measures of a tendency to deposit harmful cholesterol in walls of arteries. LDL and VLDL together usually account for about 80% of total blood cholesterol.

Blood cholesterol levels should be measured routinely for precaution and early diagnosis, only in people with other risk factor the coronary heart disease like people with high blood pressure or with diabetes or those who smoke or people with a family history of coronary heart disease.

HDL is substantially increased by exercise, by avoiding smoking, and by drinking alcohol in moderation. Total blood cholesterol can be reduced by changing diet programme and by eating less fat. There is a huge difference in the response of blood cholesterol to charges in fat intake and by doing exercise. Some people get a large fall in blood cholesterol after fairly small reduction in fat intake and increase in exercise, others get very small changes despite hectic efforts. Reduction of blood cholesterol by diet alone may be a nuisance, but has no important side-effects. A large majority of people would undoubtedly benefit from a better balance between energy intake and energy output and by substantial reduction in their intake of fats and oils.

■

Chapter 15

Long-term Complications

Today many people are concerned about their health. They find it less frightening to know what might happen, how to prevent it and how to recognize it. If the blood flows through a artery at a higher pressure the artery walls can cope with two ways: the walls of the artery may be damaged with pieces breaking off which block the artery or its tapered outlet or whole artery may burst. This 'blocking effect' and 'bursting effect' are simplification of the actual complicated processes. Arteries are usually elastic enough to cope with very high pressure indeed, they are sustained only for an hour or two of exertion. The blocking effects of high blood pressure develop slowly, over many years. Bursting effects general occurs in the smallest arteries (arterioles) with the weakest walls.

Long term complications of high blood pressure, due to blocking and bursting effect on different parts of body are impaired.

HEART AND AORTA

Due to partial blocking of the blood vessels supplying the heart, there is pain in the front of the chest when climbing upstairs known as angina. And due to complete blockage of the blood vessels supplying the heart there is partial or complete damage of the heart muscle causes 'heart attack' or 'myocardial infarction'. Bursting effect doesn't actually mean burst heart, but heart fails to pump blood out of the left ventricle as fast as it comes into the lungs from the right ventricle and sometimes it causes acute heart failure with extreme breathlessness and a sensation of drawing.

Aorta is the largest of all the arteries in the body and most elastic. After years of high blood pressure it becomes less elastic and its lining roughened by plaque and stretches to produce a swelling (aneurysm) like a sausage-shaped balloon, specially in the upper abdomen. Blood clots may form on the roughened lining of aorta and such a clot may break loose as an embolus, which may lodge down in an artery supplying a kidney or an through artery or different parts of the body, interrupting the blood supply to a kidney or leg or any part of the body. An aortic swelling can burst if the blood pressure is very high.

BRAIN

Blood clots in the carotid artery (on both sides of the front of the neck) due to high blood pressure and it may break up into small fragments. These small fragments travel up to the brain causing giddiness, faintness or confusion lasting for a few seconds. If a blood clot of carotid artery without breaking travel intact as a large embolus up into the brain, it may completely block the supply of blood to a part of the brain, causing a stroke.

Aneurysms in the arteries of brain are small bubble—like distensions of the artery wall. If a surface aneurysm bursts it release blood which bathes the brain, causing very severe headache. If an inferior aneurysm burst; it usually destroys a part of the brain, with one side paralysis.

LEGS AND FEET

Partial blockage of the artery of lower part may cause pain in the calf while walking up stairs and complete blockage causes gangrene of the toes or foot.

EYES

People with high blood pressure are more likely to develop retinal detachment, obstructed veins in the eye or obstructed arterial circulation in the eye. At very high blood pressure fluid begins to leak from arterioles into retina, causing blurred vision and visible evidence of serious risk of brain hemorrhage or permanent blindness.

KIDNEYS

At very high blood pressure the smallest arteries called as capillaries in the kidney begin to burst due to bursting effect, resulting in rapid but still reversible loss of kidney function. However, after months or years eventually, it leads to irreversible kidney failure.

OTHER PARTS OF THE BODY

Virtually any organ in the body can have its blood supply stopped by blocking effect or bursting effect and can cause internal bleeding due to high blood pressure, but serious effects are rare.

ANGINA

Angina literally means "A chocking sensation of the chest". Any pain in the middle of the front of the chest (not necessarily at all severe) which comes on with exertion and is quickly relieved by rest is likely to be anginal pain. The pain often goes down into arm or your jaw. Anginal pain rarely last longer than 5 minutes. Angina is the heart's way of saying that it is not getting enough oxygen. It is because branches of coronary arteries (the arteries that supply blood to the heart) are blocked or because heart is being overworked and therefore need more oxygen.

One of the main reason of angina is hardening and narrowing of the coronary arteries due to long history of high blood pressure. High blood pressure itself is also an immediate cause of angina. Angina is caused by excessive demands of the blood by the heart muscle. Anything which reduces this supply or increase the demand is likely to cause pain. So cold weather which requires more work from your body just to keep warm reduces the threshold for angina, and so does a big meal, requiring a big shift of blood to the intestine in order to digest it. Different types of angina are:

- **Stable or Classic angina**: This type of angina is triggered by exertion and recedes with rest. It is the most common type.
- **Unstable angina**: It is a more acute condition. It occurs unpredictably, during rest. It should be interpreted as a warning sign of more serious heart trouble.
- **Variant angina**: It is a rare type of angina. It is most often seen in women. It involves spasm of coronary artery.

People with angina can live with it comfortably, by doing little adjustment like wrap up warmly in cold weather or eat smaller meals at frequent infervals.

Angina is generally detected by Electro-Cardiogram (ECG). ECG is performed when you were at rest. Angina generally causes some changes in ECG. Angina is also detected by coronary angiography in which a dye is injected into bloodstream and then calculate the time which dye takes to reach coronary arteries.

There are plenty of drugs available for angina. By using some or all of them and with sensible changes in their lifestyle, the majority of people with angina can get along with very little chest pain. Chest pain that is not relieved within 15 minutes is likely to be caused by a coronary heart attack, not by angina.

Prevention

Exercise regularly. People who exercise are less likely to be overweight and less likely to develop angina.

- Eat a low fat and low cholesterol diet that will keep arteries free of cholesterol deposit
- Quit smoking
- Learn to control emotions. People who suppress stress are more likely to develop angina

HEART ATTACK

If angina attacks become more frequent, more severe and brought on by less exertion over a period of a week or two, this

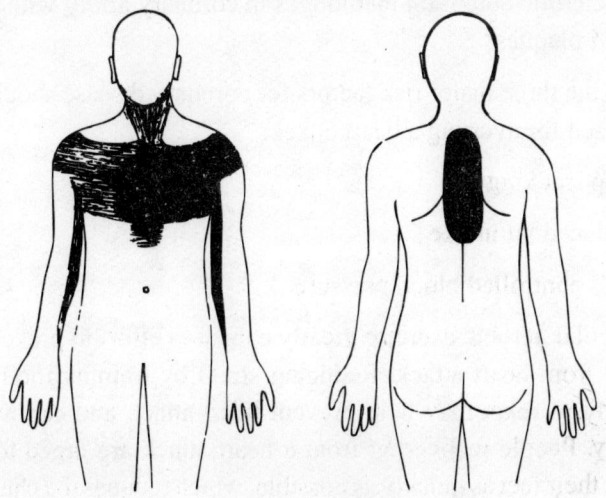

Fig. 40: Heart Attack

may indicate an imminent heart attack. The pain of a heart attack is likely to be more or less the same as of angina, perhaps more severe, but always much more persistent. Most heart attacks last longer than 5 minutes. People with long standing angina have a greater risk of developing a heart attack.

When one of the coronary arteries (which supply blood to the heart) or its branches shut down, a portion of the heart is starved of oxygen and fuel, this condition is known as **ischemia**. If an ischemic attack lasts too long, the starved heart tissue dies. This event defines heart attack—literally death of heart muscle.

The heart attack produces a prolong crushing, squeezing or burning pain in the center of the chest. The pain may radiate to the neck, to one or both the arms or the jaw. Other signs of heart attack are shortness of breath, dizziness, nausea, sweating, weak pulse, cold and damp skin, sometimes faintness and in some cases there are no symptoms.

Major risk factors for heart attack are high blood pressure, high cholesterol, smoking, stress, alcohol and a sedentary lifestyle—Most heart attacks are the end result of coronary heart disease, a atherosclerotic condition that lodges in coronary artery with fatty calcified plaques.

All the three major risk factors for coronary disease should be minimized for averting a heart attack:

- Stop smoking
- Reduced fat intake
- Well controlled blood pressure

Regular aerobic exercise greatly enhances effort to prevent or recover from heart attack. Reducing stress by training the mind and body to relax may help prevent heart attack and can aid in recovery. People recovering from a heart attack are urged to get back on their feet as quickly as possible, which reduces the chances of blood clots forming in the deep veins of the leg; the clots travel through the circulatory system and may create a blockage.

Prevention

- Make appropriate changes in diet and lifestyle
- Try to live a stress free life
- Individuals under high risk group for heart disease should have their tests done regularly

STROKE

When the blood supply to the brain is disturbed for any reason, this disorder is knows as stroke. Disruption of blood circulation to the brain are usually have drastic consequences. It occurs in two basic form and both potentially life threatening.

- Clot stroke
- Bleeding stroke or cerebral hemorrhage

About three quarters of all stroke are due to clot stroke. Blockage of the blood flowing to the brain causes clot stroke. Small fragments of clot detached from cholesterol plaque, these fragments (micro-emboli) can travel up into brain and the retina causing temporary symptoms. Some of these symptoms are disturbed vision or blindness, loss of speech, sudden loss of balance with vomiting, nausea, weakness of one side of the face or one hand or one leg and sometimes partial or complete loss of consciousness. These losses of function are called transient ischemic attacks or TIAs. None of these symptoms last for more than a few seconds or perhaps minutes. TIAs are warning symptoms of stroke. Clot stroke is often preceded by transient ischemic attack, when the interruption of blood flow lasts long enough to kill brain cells, then it produces irreversible neurological damage.

Bleeding stroke or cerebral hemorrhage occurs when an aneurysm rupture or when a weakened blood vessel in the brain starts to leak. Collection of blood into brain builds up pressure may either kill the tissue directly or destroy cells by impeding normal circulation. This type of stroke produces sudden and severe excruciating headache followed rapidly by loss of consciousness. Massive bleeding strokes are generally fatal about 80% of time.

Men are more prone for stroke than women. The main risk factors for stroke are high blood pressure, high cholesterol level, diabetes, stress a sedentary lifestyle, obesity, smoking, abuse of some stimulating drugs and birth control pills. High blood pressure is only one of the cause of stroke, but it is most important cause. If one is already suffering from high blood pressure then it is important to have the blood pressure checked and controlled. Quit smoking for preventing stroke. On the other hand people who eat a lot of vegetables and fresh fruits are much less likely to get strokes.

Stroke victims are immediately given medication to prevent further brain damage. When patient recovers from critical phase of stroke, doctor carefully reviews the patient for recovery and for prevention of future episodes of stroke. Apart from diet and life style changes, rehabilitation is the main element. Intensive rehabilitative therapy basically aims to enhance the brain's own recovery efforts, it involves speech, physical and occupational therapy.

Prevention

Adopt healthy lifestyle include eating foods that are low in fat, cholesterol and salt.

- Exercise regularly
- Quit smoking
- Monitoring and controlling blood pressure and cholesterol level
- Controlling weight